the fast 800 treats recipe book

Healthy and delicious bakes, savoury snacks and desserts for everyone to enjoy

DR CLARE BAILEY
and KATHRYN BRUTON

Foreword by DR MICHAEL MOSLEY

An Hachette UK Company
First published in Great Britain in 2024
by Short Books, an imprint of
Octopus Publishing Group Limited
Carmelite House
50 Victoria Embankment
London
EC4Y 0DZ
www.hachette.co.uk
www.octopusbooks.co.uk

Distributed in the US by
Hachette Book Group
1290 Avenue of the Americas
4th and 5th Floors
New York, NY 10104

Distributed in Canada by
Canadian Manda Group
664 Annette St.
Toronto, Ontario, Canada M6S 2GB

Recipe writer: Kathryn Bruton
Recipe tester: Caroline Barton
Nutritional analysis: Fiona Hunter
Project editor: Jo Roberts-Miller
Design and art direction: Smith & Gilmour
Photography: Smith & Gilmour
Author photographs: Lezli+Rose
Food styling: Phil Mundy
Cover design: Smith & Gilmour
Hand model: Lily Smith
Production: Emily Noto
Publisher: Joanna Copestick
Commissioning Editor: Helena Sutcliffe

ISBN: 9781780726328

A GIP catalogue record for this book is available from the
British Library.

10 9 8 7 6 5 4 3 2 1

Contents

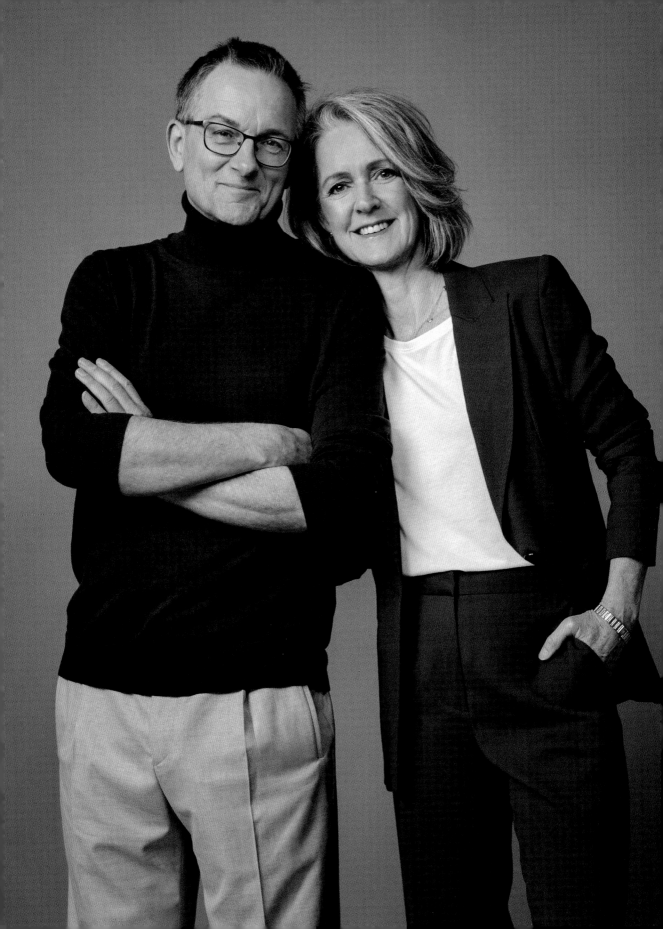

Foreword by Dr Michael Mosley

When I first met Clare at medical school in the 1980s, I was slim and athletic. This, in retrospect, is surprising since I had a terrible diet, consisting mainly of pink salami sandwiches and sugary snacks. Slowly, over the years, though, she has helped shape my tastes and what I consume, so that these days we largely eat a Mediterranean-style diet with lots of veg and oily fish.

But I am a slow learner with a very sweet tooth, so although I began eating more healthily after meeting Clare, I also continued snacking, often in secret. Crisps, biscuits, chocolates and then more biscuits. Not surprisingly, I steadily put on a lot of weight and because it was so gradual, I don't think that either Clare or I really noticed (although she did notice that I was beginning to snore, very loudly).

It wasn't until I was diagnosed with Type 2 diabetes in 2012 that I realised I was snacking my way to an early grave and that I had to do something about it. By that point, I had become a television presenter, so I decided it would be a good idea to make a documentary called *Eat, Fast and Live Longer*, where I would try to reverse my diabetes, something I was told was impossible. In the course of making that documentary, I met researchers studying intermittent fasting, invented the 5:2 diet and lost 9kg, which was enough to shrink my waist by 11cm and get my blood sugars back down to normal. I later met Professor Roy Taylor, from Newcastle University, who explained that the reason I'd developed diabetes was because I was carrying too much fat around my waist, which had infiltrated my liver and pancreas. By shedding 9kg, fast, I had got rid of that fat and my pancreas had sprung back to life. With his support I went on to write a book called *The Fast 800*, which Clare and I, and other doctors, later turned into the very popular Fast 800 online programme.

Although I understood the link between unhealthy snacking, weight gain and Type 2 diabetes, I never managed to fully shake off my addiction to sugary junk food, and for many years continued to reach for biscuits or chocolate, particularly when bored or stressed.

Fortunately, Clare decided 'If you can't beat them, join them' and started to create healthy treats, which she would offer me instead of the mass-manufactured, ultra-processed junk I craved. Food manufacturers spend huge amounts of money creating foods that are not only high in salt, fat and sugar, but finely tuned so that once you start eating them you just can't stop (or, at least, I can't).

Which is why I think what Clare has done in this book is so important. It is for those of us who want the occasional treat, but who want that treat to be as healthy as possible. It is for those of us who want to make treats we can offer to family and guests on special occasions, and not feel bad about doing so. And it is for those of us who like the idea that by making our own treats we are fighting back, in a modest way, against the giant multinationals who have done so much, down the years, to make us fat.

And, most importantly of all, these treats are delicious without inducing terrible cravings, so I hope you enjoy them. I certainly do.

Introduction by Dr Clare Bailey

This book is not about weight loss, although it may help you on your journey; it's about celebrating and savouring indulgent and satisfying healthy treats. I have often been asked to produce such a book, so am thrilled to be able to share it with you. The recipes are designed to be easy and fun to prepare, using ingredients that won't break the bank. Whether sweet or savoury, my hope is that every treat will be a joy to make, eat and share with all the family.

So, what do I mean by 'treat'? A good treat in my view should be something exciting, desirable and indulgent – something a bit special that you don't expect to have routinely. We all need treats – for celebrations, fun and a sense of delight. They get a lot of bad press, though, and many people see them as a guilty pleasure to be avoided. But I would suggest that a treat doesn't have to be something that adversely effects your health, upsets the bugs in your gut, or negatively impacts concentration, mood and learning, particularly in children. The 'treats' that have those effects are likely to be ultra-processed foods (UPF) – all of which are high in poor-quality ingredients and low in important nutrients, such as protein and fibre (both key in helping us to feel comfortably full after eating).

With the help of the brilliant food writer Kathryn Bruton, I have carefully researched and created recipes that are made with natural and healthy ingredients, so you don't need to worry or feel guilty about enjoying them. These treats can be enjoyed without counting calories, in the knowledge that they won't significantly spike your blood sugars. However, for anyone doing an 800–1000 calorie fast day, I have provided the calorie information below each recipe so you can keep track.

If, like Michael, you find sweet things irresistible, switching to these delicious healthy alternatives will decrease your sweet tooth and down-regulate your cravings over time. With adults and children now eating over 50% of their food in the form of UPFs, it's increasingly important to embrace a healthy approach, particularly when cooking for young children. So, with your future health and that of your family in mind, I have set out to show that we can all enjoy fabulous, nutritious and varied treats that are suitable for all. Many are also easy for children to make, such as the Strawberry and Cream Ice Pops (page 172) or the Chocolate Fruit Kebabs (page 154).

When our son was 18 months old, he tasted chocolate for the first time at an Easter celebration and chanted 'More chocolate, more chocolate!' all the way home. It's no surprise that some sweet and starchy foods, often combined with poor-quality fats, have a particular allure that makes them almost addictive. They are designed simply to make you go on eating. Most of us don't need more added sugar, and that particularly applies to children. Once they get a taste for sweet things it can be a challenge to re-set but the benefits of doing so are huge. We all need treats and indulgences, but it doesn't need to be a sugar fest that sends your blood sugars soaring and ends up stored as fat. With so much temptation at every turn, from the corner shop to major supermarkets, we need to be aware that avoiding a sweet tooth almost certainly starts in pregnancy and even pre-conception. So when it comes to children, they just don't need all that sugar, starch and those unidentifiable ingredients in the UPFs. And, if they don't have access to it, they won't miss it. Of course, you can work to re-set a preference for sweet things, but it's better to start early!

As I will show you, it is possible to produce delicious treats that still give you that satisfying pleasure hit – such as ice creams, cakes and biscuits, comforting fruit puddings and chocolate bakes – without harming your health. And it really doesn't mean turning into the Grinch. With a few swaps and carefully chosen fruit for flavour and sweetness, you can savour those delicious indulgences and enjoy all your favourite desserts – from Chocolate Chip Banana Bread (page 117) to Apple Crumble (page 126).

With recipes for every occasion that won't sabotage a diet, there are treats for when you need an energy boost without a sugar high and for your children to take to school without having a sugar rush followed by a crash. They may even be able to brag that they made the treats themselves, as many of the recipes are very simple! The more children are involved in cooking with you, the better their connection with the ingredients and the more likely they will be to enjoy these lovely, healthy treats. Most of the recipes are also packed full of protein and fibre, so you feel comfortably satiated without the need to keep reaching for more.

After more than 30 years as a GP, I've found it incredibly rewarding to see a move away from automatically prescribing escalating amounts of medication to patients with metabolic diseases such as Type 2 diabetes, hypertension and those living with obesity and the myriad complications and chronic diseases associated with it. Thankfully so many conditions can now be prevented and reversed with the right lifestyle support. Following the best evidence and our previous books, the Fast 800 team have contributed to helping hundreds of thousands of people turn their health and lives around. Thank you to so many of you for sharing your incredible, inspiring and touching stories. We love to hear them and wish you well on your journey. For more information and support see www.thefast800.com and follow me on Instagram @drclarebailey and www.parentingmatters.co.uk.

A note from Kathryn Bruton
When Clare and I first discussed the concept of this book, I was excited at the prospect of creating a whole series of healthy treats, desserts and indulgent snacks. For each recipe, we have carefully chosen ingredients that are both delicious and healthy. Sweetness is added by using fresh fruit, dried fruit and/or very small quantities of honey or maple syrup. We opt for flours such as buckwheat, wholegrain spelt or ground almonds, rather than white flour. Unsweetened cocoa powder is used, as well as chocolate with a high cocoa content. Every recipe has been tried and tested to make sure it is simple and easy to make. You'll find adaptations of family favourites, recipes that kids will enjoy cooking as well as eating, savoury treats and much more. Some personal favourites include the creamy Three-Ingredient Chocolate Mousse (page 147), which is a fantastic recipe for entertaining; get the children involved in making the Apple and Banana Muffins with a Crumble Topping (page 67); and for those who have less of a sweet tooth, try the Savoury Parmesan Popcorn (page 98).

Treats – What to Avoid and What to Embrace

WHAT TO AVOID

1. Ultra-processed foods

Ultra-processed foods (UPFs) are foods produced in factories and typically include lots of poor-quality fats, carbs, sugar and salt. Shockingly, they now make up over 50% of the UK diet (the figure is even higher in the USA) and are linked with major health problems, including expanding waistlines, rising blood pressure, a multitude of chronic diseases, such as Type 2 diabetes, and depressed mood. They are hard to avoid, particularly when it comes to sweet things like baked goods, cakes, biscuits, sweets, crisps and breakfast cereals. Because they are high in carbs and low in important nutrients, like protein and fibre, UPFs are likely to spike blood sugars then cause them to crash, leaving you craving more. Many of these 'treats' are designed to keep you wanting more – they bypass your body's hormones that tell you when you are full, so you just go on eating. And that is how they get us hooked!

One of the worst consequences of eating lots of ultra-processed snacks is the impact they have on our gut microbiome, particularly on all the 'good' microbes that influence the body's processes in ways we are only just beginning to understand. These microorganisms depend on us to provide them with good-quality fibre, which they use to produce vital chemicals to reduce inflammation in the body, protect our immune system and generally keep us healthy, as well as producing our own natural antidepressants, including serotonin.

And that is not the end of the story. UPFs also contain synthetic substances which neither we, nor our microbes, have been exposed to before, such as hydrogenated fats and emulsifiers, which give junk food a smooth texture and stop them from going off. Many also contain chemicals for carbonating, firming, bulking and anti-bulking, de-foaming, anti-caking and glazing, not to mention sequestrants and humectants. These chemicals contribute to gut and metabolic disease through alterations to the gut microbiome, damaging our intestinal mucus layer and driving inflammatory responses.

So how can you spot an ultra-processed food? It will probably be heavily packaged and heavily promoted. Read the label – there will be a multitude of industrial substances that you would never find in your kitchen and additives to make the food difficult to resist. If there are five or more ingredients, and those ingredients include numbers or have names you don't recognise, the chances are it's ultra-processed.

2. Sugar and sweeteners

Whether it is brown or white, granulated or caster – we know about the dangers of sugar. The natural sugars you find in fruits, such as dates, figs and apricots, are far better for us because they come bound in fibre and packed with health-promoting phytonutrients. That's why eating an apple, peel and all, is much better for you than drinking apple juice, where the fibre and most of the goodness have been removed. The fibre you find in fruit also supports a healthy gut microbiome. Dried fruit contains more sugar by weight than fresh fruit, but relatively small amounts bring both sweetness and flavour. As far as possible, we have used fruit to add a touch of sweetness to our recipes. We occasionally include a little natural honey or maple syrup, but these ingredients do at least include some other healthy nutrients (unlike sugar!).

Not surprisingly, the simplest way to reduce sugar in your diet is to cook your food from scratch – that way you know exactly what goes into it. The 'hidden' sugars in ready-made convenience foods can be very hard to spot.

If the word 'sugar' does not appear in the ingredients list, look for alternative names, such as maltose, dextrose, fructose, glucose and lactose. There are more than 60 different names for what is essentially sugar, and these can add up to being the main ingredient!

Artificial sweeteners are another challenge. They are many times sweeter than sugar, which can increase sugar cravings, and there is evidence that some artificial sweeteners can damage the good microbes in your gut. If you do want to use a sweetener, I'd recommend stevia, which is based on a South American plant. Once you start making the recipes in this book, though, you'll find your tastes change and, as your palate adapts, you won't miss the sugar.

3. Processed carbohydrates

Most ultra-processed pastries, snacks, puddings and breakfast cereals are made from white flour, which is low in nutrients. Instead, we want to encourage you to embrace healthier, tastier, more nutritious 'complex' carbs, such as wholegrain flours, rolled oats and quinoa, as they contain much more protein, fibre and nutrients.

We include a variety of accessible wholegrains in our recipes that should be available in most large supermarkets, such as wholegrain spelt (an ancient grain which contains the nutritious bran – germ and all) or buckwheat (which is actually a seed, making it gluten free, and which has a slightly nutty taste and behaves almost like flour). To keep it simple we've chosen a small selection of healthy grains for the recipes. This will allow you to get used to just a few different varieties at first. We have also replaced processed white flour with ground almonds, which has a grainier texture and firmer consistency, making it ideal for desserts like our Nutty Chocolate Orange Fridge Brownies (page 42) and Orange and Pistachio Upside-down Cake

(page 110). It also contains far more nutrients, protein and fibre. It doesn't act like a classic cake batter, though, so don't expect the fluffy consistency of a Victoria sponge.

And, if you like porridge, instead of buying ready-made sachets of instant oats that will spike your blood sugars, go for rolled whole oats that take a bit longer to cook but are slow release thanks to that extra fibre and which leave you feeling full for longer.

WHAT TO EMBRACE
1. Protein

Protein is key! We recommend eating well above the current government guidelines, which is 45g protein a day for women and 55g for men. It is clear, for example, that women going through the menopause and older adults need more than that as we process proteins less effectively as we age.

If you don't get enough protein in your diet, you will feel hungry much of the time. That's because protein is one of the main drivers of appetite and plays a vital role in cell repair, maintaining muscles, feeding a healthy immune system and much more. Research shows that simply by increasing protein intake from 15% to 30% of daily calories, overweight women ate 441 fewer calories each day – without intentionally restricting anything. Another study, this time involving overweight adolescent girls, showed that having a high-protein breakfast reduced cravings and late-night snacking. And if you need any more convincing about the importance of protein, in a 12-month study, the high-protein group in 130 overweight people on a calorie-restricted diet lost 53% more body fat than a normal-protein group eating the same number of calories.

If you are on an 800–1000 calorie fast day, aim for at least 50–60g protein and try to spread it across your meals. Michael and

I love eggs for breakfast and, although people used to worry about cholesterol in eggs, the research shows that from a health point of view they are either neutral or beneficial. So, we are happily eating a couple of eggs most days. Other rich sources of protein include meat (typically 30g protein per 100g), fish (22g per 100g), lentils (9g per 100g) and tofu (8g per 100g).

2. Fibre

It's worth saying again that most of us don't get even half of the daily fibre we need (30g a day). We know that eating plenty of fibre will help keep our bowels 'regular', but fibre also brings other benefits, including lowering cholesterol levels and maintaining a healthy weight, as well as helping to control blood sugar levels. Fibre is also essential for feeding your microbiome, those all-important bugs in your gut. Keep them happy and healthy and they, in turn, will look after you! This is why so many of the recipes are relatively high in fibre, such as the High-fibre Carrot and Pecan Muffins (page 64) and the Mango and Lime Chia Pots (page 141).

3. Healthy fats and dairy

A healthy, Mediterranean-style diet contains plenty of 'good' fats, such as olive oil, groundnut oil (peanut oil), avocado oil, oily fish, nuts and seeds, all of which have been shown to lower your risk of stroke and heart disease. We've included nuts in many of our Fast 800 treats as they are such a great nutritional boost.

When it comes to dairy products, such as yoghurt, cheese, milk and butter – all part of the Mediterranean-style diet – the latest research suggests that full-fat is best as it's minimally processed and less likely to lead to weight gain or Type 2 diabetes. Unlike starchy carbohydrates, natural fats are very important for absorbing fat-soluble vitamins. They are also an excellent source of slow-burn energy and won't spike your blood sugar levels.

Michael and I love full-fat Greek yoghurt; we eat it for breakfast with fruit and nuts, or dolloped on a pudding or drizzled over fresh fruit. Check the label to make sure it doesn't contain the starchy thickeners, sugars or sweeteners that are often added to enhance low-fat products – particularly the more processed fruit yoghurts. We would encourage you to enjoy full-fat yoghurt, milk and cheese, in moderation, as part of a healthy Mediterranean style-diet.

4. Fruit

Fruit contains lots of health-promoting phytonutrients and fibre, which are concentrated in the skin. So do eat your fruit whole, preferably not peeled or juiced as this reduces the fibre. Ideally go for berries and hard fruits, such as pears and apples, that have a lower sugar content, rather than sweet tropical varieties, such as melons or grapes. Aim for one or two portions a day and, to make this easier to achieve, keep tinned fruit in the cupboard (make sure it's stored in fruit juice, not syrup) and diced rhubarb, chopped apples or a bag of frozen berries in the freezer, so that they are readily available to warm up in the microwave. Frozen or tinned fruits are just as healthy and often fresher as they are tinned or frozen soon after picking. And using a microwave is a quick, efficient and safe way to defrost fruit (and veg).

Fruit is best eaten either with a meal or straight after a meal, rather than as a snack. If you really need a snack, go for a small handful of nuts or seeds, a piece of cheese or perhaps a Pistachio and Cranberry Bliss Ball (page 49), a Chocolate Raspberry Nutty Bite (page 176) or some Savoury Trail Mix (page 37).

The Fast 800 Programme – a Recap

You don't have to be following the Fast 800 programme to use this book. These recipes are for anyone who enjoys a healthy home-made treat. They are simple, tasty, relatively low-sugar and child-friendly recipes that are easy and fun to make, while also being indulgent. No calorie counting needs to be involved.

But if you are doing, have done, or plan to do the Fast 800, or simply wish to embark on a re-set, these new treats are also for you. The Fast 800 is a carefully researched, flexible, three-stage weight-loss programme that starts with rapid weight loss to kick-start fat-burning, moves on to intermittent fasting and finishes with what we call The Way of Life.

STAGE 1
RAPID WEIGHT LOSS

This approach involves both calorie and carbohydrate restriction, and is for those who want or need to lose weight fast; it involves sticking to around 800–1000 calories a day, and eating two big or three smaller meals. The food is based on a Mediterranean-style diet, where carbohydrates are kept fairly low, but not very low. This phase of the diet is not suitable for everyone – see page 12 for further information.

During the initial, rapid weight-loss phase you will cut right back on sweet and starchy carbs, as these stop you going into ketosis. However, on days when you are feeling hungry, you can choose from a range of top-ups to take your daily quota up to 1000 calories (page 186). You can stay in Stage 1 for anything from three to 12 weeks, before easing into Stage 2. That said, many people skip Stage 1 and go straight to Stage 2.

STAGE 2
INTERMITTENT FASTING

During this stage, you will continue to lose weight steadily, but at a slightly slower rate. You pick two, three or four days each week, when you stick to 800–1000 calories, still keeping carbohydrates to a minimum (as on Stage 1), while for the rest of the week you follow a lowish-carb Mediterranean-style diet not counting calories.

People who've done our online course say they often start the Intermittent Fasting (IF) by following a 3:4 pattern (not worrying about calories on Friday and at weekends, and restricting themselves to 800–1000 calories for the remaining four days). They may then move to the 5:2 pattern, eating healthily five days a week and cutting calories just two days a week.

STAGE 3
THE WAY OF LIFE

This is the long-term maintenance phase, when the core principles of eating a lowish-carbohydrate diet become a way of life. Stage 3 enables you to enjoy a healthy, Mediterranean-style diet with plenty of protein (aiming for around 1g protein per kilogram of body weight), some complex carbohydrates and, of course, some healthy treats!

For a more in-depth explanation as to how to follow the Fast 800 Programme, go to www.thefast800.com. As well as providing more information and FAQs, you can access the Fast 800 programme for extra support, including recipes, shopping lists and tailored meal plans, as well as exercise, behavioural and mindfulness programmes, to help keep you on track.

Time-restricted eating (TRE)

We are fans of time-restricted eating (TRE), where you limit your eating window and extend your normal overnight fast. You might, for example, try eating your last meal at least three hours before you go to bed, and then delay breakfast until an hour or so after you wake up. If you stop eating by 8pm and don't eat again till 8am, that is a form of TRE known as 12:12. If you find that easy to do, you might want to try 14:10 or even a 16:8. TRE is something you can readily combine with the Fast 800 programme.

Exclusions and cautions

Rapid weight loss does not suit everyone. If you have a significant underlying medical condition, for example diabetes, and are on insulin or other medication; if you have high blood pressure, moderate or severe retinopathy, epilepsy, gallstones, or are pregnant or breastfeeding, please talk to your doctor before going on this diet. It is not suitable for teenagers, people with a history of an eating disorder or a psychiatric illness, or if you are unwell, underweight or doing endurance exercise. See the FAQs at www.thefast800.com for more information.

When to enjoy treats

When it comes to treats, not only does it matter how much you eat, but also when you eat and what you eat alongside your treat. Put simply, if you eat carb-rich foods on an empty stomach, you are more likely to get a rapid spike in blood sugars, quickly followed by a sugar crash that leaves you craving more. But if you eat the same amount of carbs straight after a healthy meal they will be absorbed more gradually, leading to a lower spike. This is because the fat, fibre and protein in the meal you've just eaten will flatten the glucose curve and allow a slower release of glucose into your bloodstream.

What time of day you eat your treat also matters. Studies have shown that food eaten later at night, within three hours of going to bed, is more likely to end up being stored as fat than a similar snack eaten earlier in the day.

Eating late at night is also more likely to lead to acid reflux and disrupted sleep, as your body struggles to process food when your circadian clock is telling your digestive system to close down for the night. It's a bit like going into a restaurant late at night when the staff are getting ready to close – they are not going to be happy.

Another good reason to avoid late-night snacks is that, by cutting them out, your overnight fast is extended and your gut gets a well-earned break from the hard work of digesting food. Think of your gut as being like a motorway that needs to be closed overnight for the surface to be repaired. It's only when there is no late-night food travelling down your digestive tract that your body can get on with the essential business of repairing the lining of your gut.

Tips for Using This Book

SYMBOLS

We have added the following symbols to the top of each page, so you can quickly spot which treats might suit you best. These are guidelines only and you should always consult your doctor if you are unsure which foods are best for you.

 These recipes either do not contain any animal-derived substances, or such ingredients are optional.

 These recipes do not contain any ingredients containing gluten (with the exception of oats, which can contain trace amounts of gluten or the protein avenin, which some people with coeliac disease cannot tolerate).

 These recipes do not contain nuts or nut products. (Check the ingredients carefully to make sure they have been packaged in a nut-free environment, though, if you are very sensitive.)

 These recipes do not contain dairy products, or have a non-dairy alternative given.

 These recipes are freezer-friendly.

 These are the quick and easy recipes for a super-speedy treat.

You will also find nutritional information below each recipe, including calories (cals), protein (g), carbs (g), sugar (g) and fibre (g) for each individual serving.

Please note – we include calorie counts as a rough guide only. There are variations between different counters and apps, so don't be too concerned by a few extra calories here or there.

Melting chocolate in the microwave

You can use a bain marie to melt chocolate, but I aways pop it in the microwave. Make sure you only heat it initially for 30 seconds, then stir the chocolate and cook it in bursts of 15 seconds, checking after each burst, to avoid overheating, otherwise the chocolate will stiffen and burn.

Non-dairy milk and yoghurt alternatives

Where we recommend using full-fat Greek yoghurt, please feel free to swap for a thick dairy-free alternative. These may not contain the same level of protein, though. Similarly, replace full-fat milk with a non-dairy equivalent and, in most cases, butter can be replaced with coconut oil.

Eggs

I always use free-range eggs. Not only are these a higher welfare choice, they also contain more omega-3 than the factory-farmed equivalent.

Gluten-free flours

Unfortunately, gluten-free flours do not always behave the same as flours with gluten, so it isn't always a straightforward swap. For this reason, we've tried to include as many recipes as possible that contain ground almonds or buckwheat flour, which are naturally gluten free.

What about salt?

I have only included salt as part of the recipe in a small number of treats. However, I find that adding a pinch of salt when mixing the batter can really enhance the natural flavour of a biscuit or cake, particularly when cooking with chocolate or nuts. When I bake with butter, I always use salted butter, for the same reason. If you prefer less salt, or need to avoid it for medical reasons, feel free to omit as you wish.

FAQs

Can the recipes be enjoyed by people who aren't following the Fast 800 diet?

These treats are for anyone who wants to avoid mass-produced, ultra-processed foods and, instead, enjoy delicious, healthy treats that are suitable for all the family. Not only are they free of the artificial ingredients you find in factory-produced foods, but they will satisfy rather than feed your sugar cravings. However, they are also ideal for anyone doing the Fast 800 diet, so if you need to look at the nutritional information, you will find it below each recipe. We all need a treat at times, whether sweet or savoury!

Are the recipes gluten free, dairy free and vegan friendly?

To make it easier to identify specific recipes for people with dietary requirements, we have included symbols to show when a recipe is vegan, gluten free,* nut free, dairy free or when it is freezable or quick to make. For the vast majority of the dairy recipes, a swap to a lactose free or vegan equivalent should work fine (we often suggest using coconut yoghurt or cream instead). *For recipes containing oats, in Australia and New Zealand, oats are not designated as gluten free. Those with coeliac disease should check with their medical specialists before consuming products containing oats.

Can I enjoy these treats with children?

These recipes have been created for families and with children in mind. The treats are indulgent and fun (see page 39 for Chocolate Pennies, or page 68 for Throw-it-all-together Blueberry and Ginger Muffins), but they are much lower in sugar than commercial products. The more you can keep children away from the allure of ultra-sweet sugary 'treats', the better. If your children are already craving sugary things, by adapting these recipes and adding extra honey, for example, you can appeal to their tastes, but then gradually reduce the sweetness and sugar content. This may take weeks, but is so worth it!

If you have children I would encourage you to cook with them from a young age, so they are familiar with different foods, textures and flavours to help reduce fussy eating. Children are naturally conservative and it can take many trials before they accept new foods. On the whole kids love to be involved and to help. The more you explore and celebrate different foods, the better. Cooking together helps to build relationships, as well as helping your child become capable and confident. Unfortunately, most children grow up surrounded by sweet temptations. Many of these heathy recipes, such as the Super Seeded Flapjacks (page 29) or Chocolate Almond Fridge Bars (page 45) , would work well in a lunch box, or simply as a pleasing alternative to an ultra-processed snack.

Are the recipes expensive?

We have done our best to ensure that our recipes are both affordable and accessible, so you are not trailing around looking for obscure ingredients that break the bank. They should all be available from most supermarkets. Having the right foods at hand means you are less likely to nip round the corner to the convenience store for a bar of chocolate or a sugary snack, so keep frozen, tinned and jarred ingredients stocked up. If you are prepared, when you feel the urge for a cookie or for a quick pudding, you'll have the dried, tinned or frozen fruit to hand for things like Easy Fig and Cinnamon Cookies (page 22), Quick Baked Pears with Ginger and Walnuts (page 105) or Chocolate Raspberry Nutty Bites (page 176).

Is it true that I can't eat fruit-based treats if I'm following a keto diet?

Typical keto diets are very low in carbohydrates, making it hard to include much or any fruit. Because the Fast 800 means you reduce calories as well as sugary carbs, you can be less restrictive about carbs and still achieve ketosis, which is why lots of our recipes, such as Ginger Roasted Rhubarb with Nut Crumble (page 118) and Raspberry, Peach and Chocolate Cupcakes (page 52), contain fruit.

How do I avoid the temptation to grab a processed snack instead?

This can be difficult if you are surrounded by ultra-processed snacks at home, in the office or when you are out and about. Where possible, ask your work colleagues to keep them out of sight or further away. Also try telling them about your healthy changes – you might even find they want to join you. Be prepared for temptations and have healthy alternatives, such as Iced Apricot and Orange Cupcakes (page 57) or a handful of nuts, available instead.

Can the treats be frozen?

Almost all of these treats can be frozen, so you can cook batches and pop them in the freezer ready to enjoy at your leisure. Make sure any hot food has been cooled first and that everything is safely wrapped or stored in a sealed container before freezing. You can also pack up your treats in smaller portions in case you want a quick snack (or two!) without defrosting the whole dish.

How do I combat sugar cravings?

We all get cravings but research shows that when you switch to healthier alternatives these cravings reduce. That said, the best time to enjoy a treat is straight after a meal. By doing this, the fat, fibre and protein in the meal cushion the release of sugar from the snack.

The food is also processed more slowly so you are not left craving more. Also, try eating slowly, as you are likely to eat less, reduce a sugar surge and get the maximum pleasure from your scrumptious treat. So, savour your Chocolate Cherry Coconut Bar (page 46) or your Apple and Peanut Butter 'Bagel' (page 34)!

Can I eat treats on a fasting day?

Yes, you can eat a snack on a fast day! But it is best eaten after a meal. Why not go for a protein-rich recipe like Almond and Plum Sponge Pudding (page 132) or a Chorizo and Parsley Muffin (page 72)?

Which kind of chocolate is best?

If you need a chocolate hit, it's always better to go for dark chocolate (over 70% cocoa solids), instead of milk or white chocolate. This is because dark chocolate contains beneficial compounds called flavanols, which have been shown to reduce inflammation and improve blood pressure. The darker the chocolate, the more flavanols it usually contains. There are none in white chocolate and very few in milk, and they have a lot more sugar! Manufacturers often process out the bitter-tasting natural cacao (where all the good stuff comes from) by adding sugar and milk. We've created recipes using dark chocolate, balancing any bitterness with other delicious flavours to give you as much goodness from the natural cocoa as possible.

What if I can't find ingredients where I live?

Most ingredients used are readily available. If you can't find any ingredients in your local supermarket (for example, stem ginger isn't widely available in Australia), they can be purchased in delis and online. For 1 ball of stem ginger or 1 tablespoon of ginger syrup, you can try substituting ½ teaspoon of ground ginger mixed with 1 tablespoon honey.

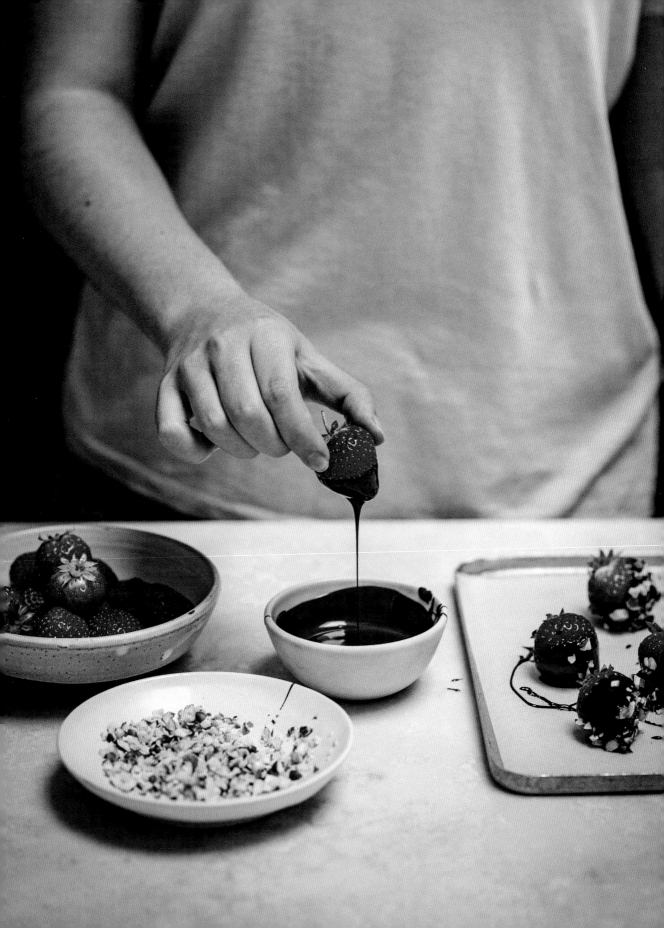

Cookies, Bars & Bites

Chocolate-dipped Strawberries with Hazelnuts

SERVES | **PREP**
2 | **5** mins

30g dark chocolate
    (at least 70%)
10 medium strawberries
20g hazelnuts, finely chopped

Jazz up your strawberries and make these colourful, chocolate-dipped, nut-speckled treats. Kids will have fun making these and devouring them too!

1. Place the chocolate in a microwave-safe bowl and microwave for 30 seconds, then in bursts of 15 seconds, stirring each time, until melted.

2. Dip one half of each strawberry into the melted chocolate, then dip in the chopped hazelnuts. Refrigerate until set. The strawberries will keep in the fridge for a couple of days.

PER SERVING / 170 CALS / PROTEIN 2.8G / SUGAR 13.1G / FIBRE 3.7G / CARBS 13.4G

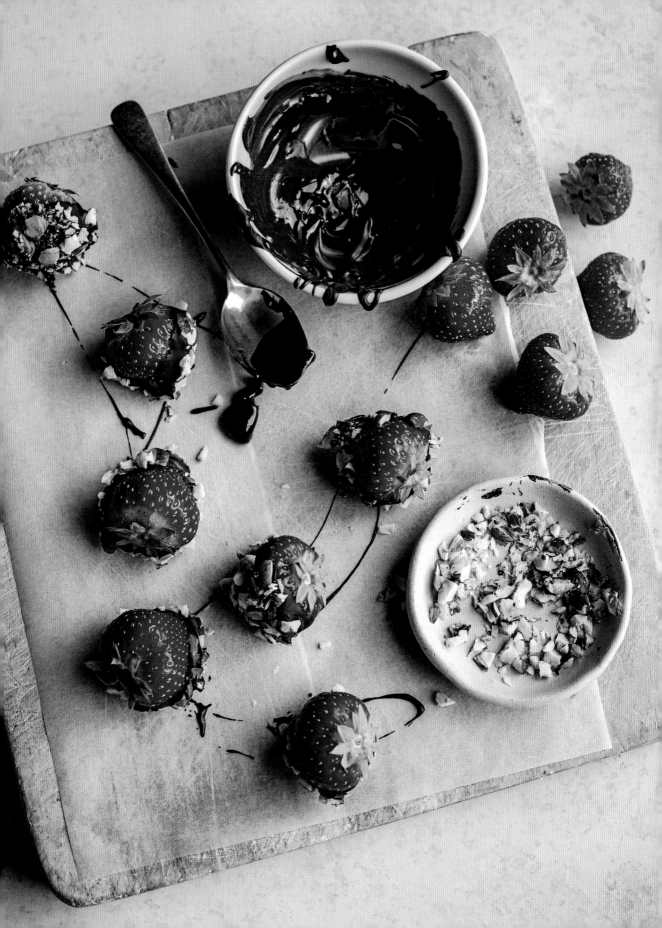

Chocolate Peanut Butter Cookies

MAKES	PREP	COOK
8	**2** mins	**12–15** mins

50g rolled oats
1 large ripe banana (or 2 small),
    peeled and mashed
2 level tsp unsweetened
    cocoa powder
2 level tbsp unsweetened
    smooth or crunchy peanut
    butter (or almond butter)
1 tbsp honey (optional)

COOK'S TIP
You can make your own
nut butter with almost any
shelled nuts by blitzing them
with a blender until they
forms a paste.

Super easy, these five-ingredient chocolate cookies are ideal for 'non-bakers' and perfect for cooking with kids. They are surprisingly high in fibre, a nutrient that most of us are lacking in, and they are also good for the gut microbiome. As a self-confessed chocoholic, Michael loves these quick and easy cookies!

1. Preheat the oven to 200°C/Fan 180°C/Gas 6 and line a baking tray with non-stick baking paper.

2. Mix all the ingredients together in a medium bowl, adding a pinch of salt.

3. Dollop the mixture on to the prepared baking tray to make 8 cookies and bake for 12–15 minutes.

4. Leave to cool on the tray.

5. Store the cookies in an airtight container.

PER SERVING / 66 CALS / PROTEIN 2.2G / SUGAR 3.2G / FIBRE 1.2G / CARBS 9G

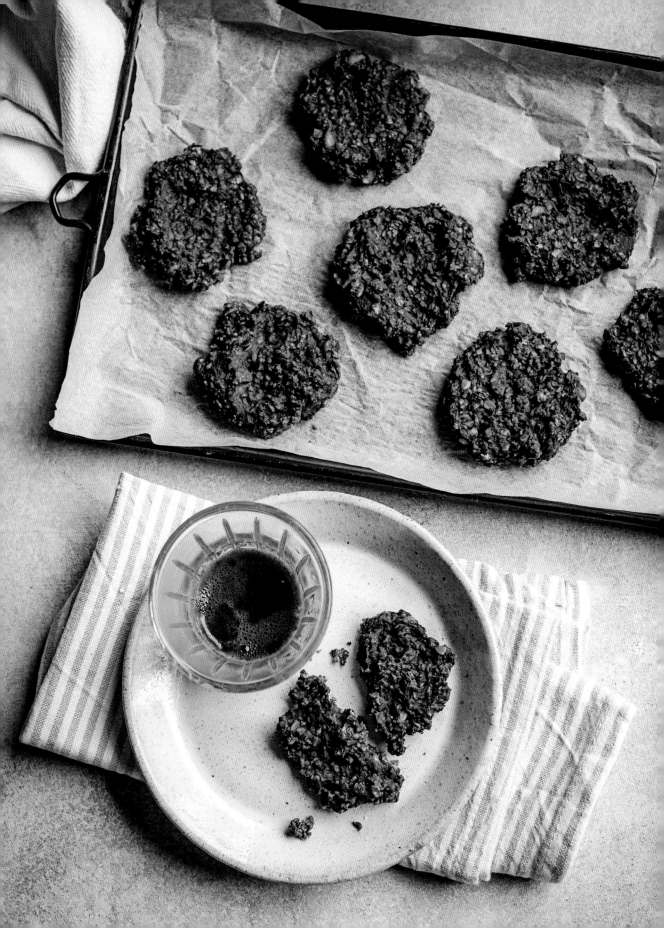

Easy Fig and Cinnamon Cookies

MAKES | **PREP** | **COOK**
12 | **10** mins | **12** mins

50g coconut oil
75g ground almonds
2 medium free-range
  egg whites
4 large dried figs, stalks
  removed and finely chopped
25g rolled oats
1 heaped tsp ground cinnamon

COOK'S TIP
Add an extra fig if you
want more sweetness.

You can whip up some of these chewy, figgy cookies in minutes, leaving plenty of time to sit and savour them. Time well spent.

1. Preheat the oven to 190°C/Fan 170°C/Gas 5 and line one baking tray with non-stick baking paper and another tray with kitchen roll.

2. Place the coconut oil, ground almonds, egg whites and half the chopped figs in a bowl and mix together using an electric whisk or blitz together with a hand-held blender.

3. Add the oats, remaining chopped figs and cinnamon to the bowl and fold into the mixture with a spoon.

4. Divide the mixture into 12 and roll each portion between your palms, then flatten into small discs. Place on the parchment-lined baking tray and bake for 12 minutes, or until golden.

5. Remove the cookies from the oven and transfer to the tray lined with kitchen roll to absorb any excess oil. Leave to cool.

6. Store in an airtight container.

PER SERVING / 96 CALS / PROTEIN 2.5G / SUGAR 1.9G / FIBRE 0.7G / CARBS 3.5G

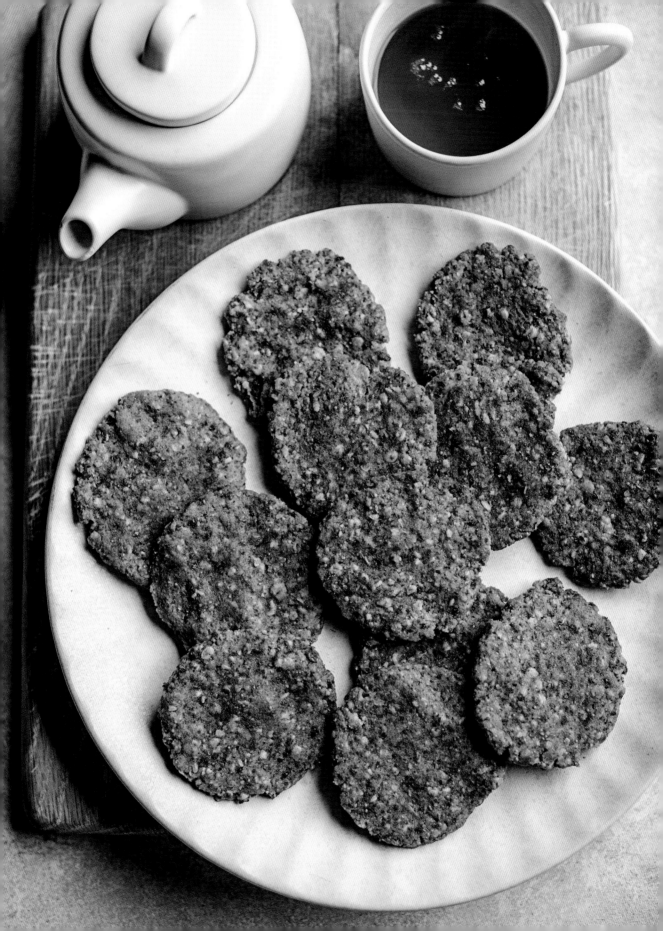

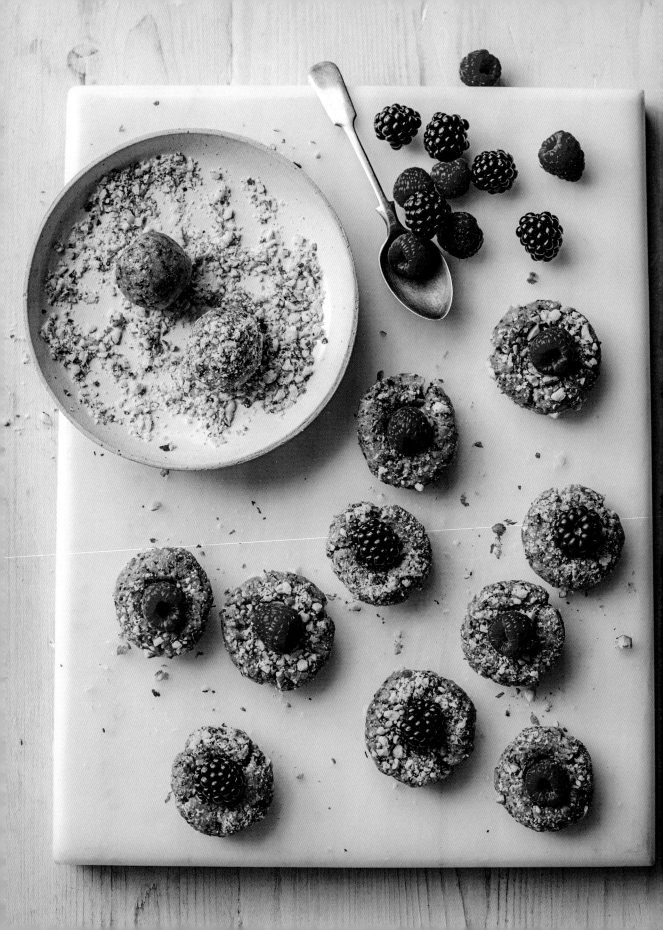

Fruity Fridge Biscuits

MAKES
12

PREP
20 mins

100g cashews
4 dried apricots, diced
1 tbsp coconut oil
2 tsp vanilla extract
1 tbsp honey (optional)
50g rolled oats
1 tbsp chia seeds
25g toasted hazelnuts, chopped
12 raspberries or blackberries,
    for decoration

These cute, colourful, fruity mouthfuls are fun to make – especially with a child – weighing ingredients, then rolling out the mixture and pressing with a little thumbprint. You could use any small pieces of fruit for decoration.

1. Place the cashews, apricots, coconut oil, vanilla extract, honey, if using, and oats in a food processor or blender and blitz to a paste, keeping some texture.

2. Add the chia seeds and blitz again briefly.

3. Divide the mixture into 12 pieces. Tightly roll each piece into a ball the size of a walnut, then roll each ball in the chopped hazelnuts to cover.

4. Transfer to a plate and gently press a thumb into the centre of each biscuit to leave a small hole. Gently press a raspberry or blackberry into each hole and refrigerate until needed.

5. Store the biscuits in an airtight container in the fridge.

PER SERVING / 101 CALS / PROTEIN 3.1G / SUGAR 3.4G / FIBRE 2.2G / CARBS 7.5G

Ginger and Cranberry Rock Cakes

MAKES **12** | **PREP** **15** mins | **COOK** **20** mins

2 medium free-range
    egg whites
50g ground almonds
50g rolled oats
50g coconut oil (or butter)
3 balls of stem ginger in syrup,
    drained and finely chopped
25g dried cranberries,
    roughly chopped

COOK'S TIP
The cooled rock cakes
can be kept in an airtight
container for up to 5 days.

These zingy ginger and cranberry rock cakes are crunchy on the outside and soft and chewy on the inside. They contain plenty of fibre, as well as protein from the nuts and eggs. Easy to make and ideal to add to a lunch box. They would also taste great crumbled into yoghurt with a handful of berries or scattered over stewed fruit.

1. Preheat the oven to 180°C/Fan 160°C/Gas 4 and line a large baking tray with non-stick baking paper.

2. Place all the ingredients, except the cranberries, in a food processor or blender and blitz briefly to combine. You can also mix vigorously by hand but the cakes may end up a little more crumbly. Stir in the cranberries.

3. Use two dessertspoons to divide the mixture into 12 pieces, scooping out the dough and dropping it on to the prepared tray. Bake for about 20 minutes or until golden brown.

4. Transfer carefully to a wire rack and leave to cool for a few minutes before serving.

———

PER SERVING / 73 CALS / PROTEIN 2.1G / SUGAR 1G / FIBRE 0.5G / CARBS 3.7G

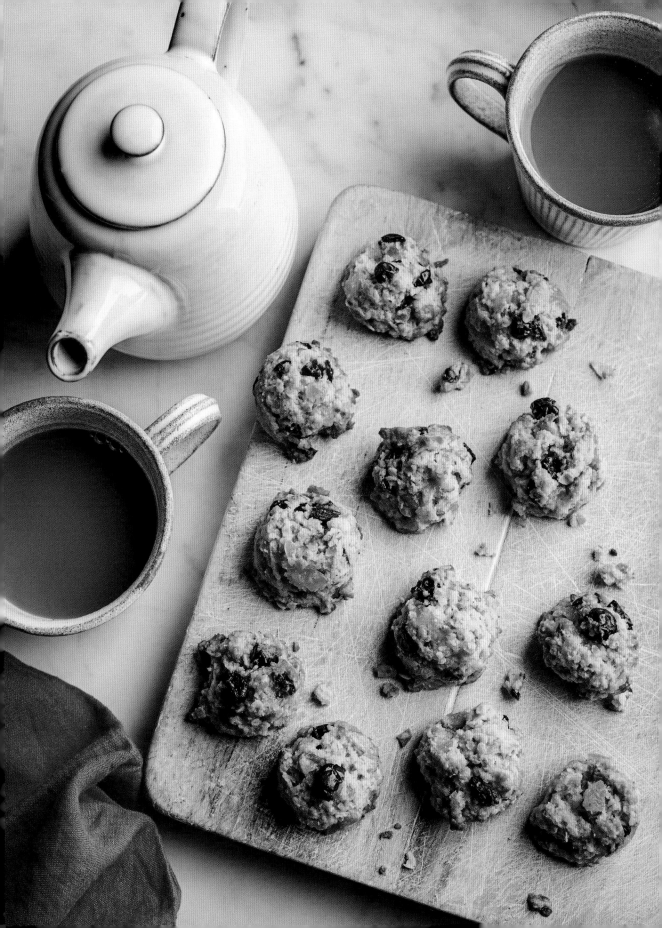

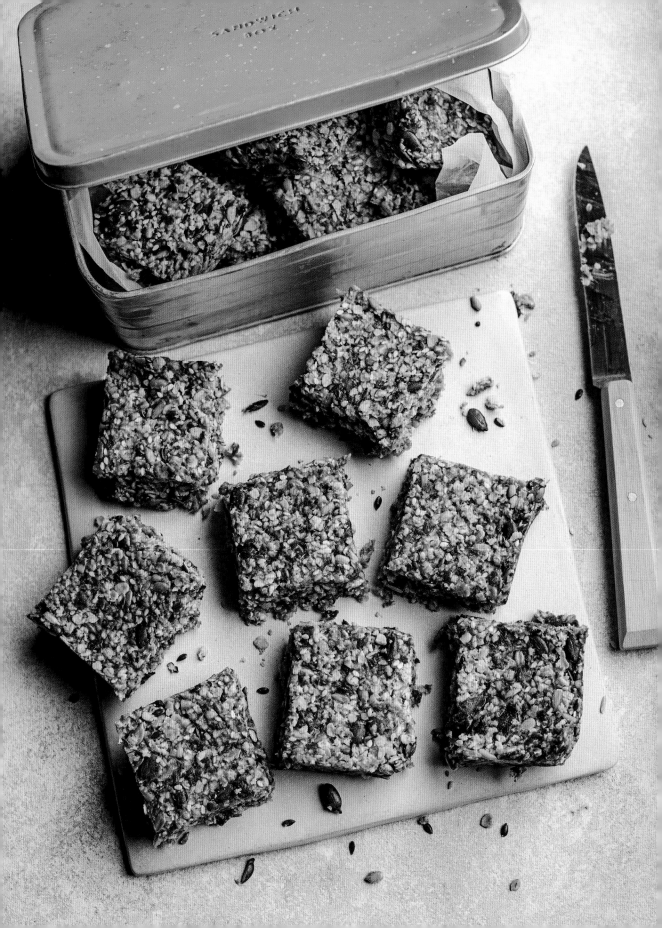

Super Seeded Flapjacks

MAKES | **PREP** | **COOK**
16 | **10** mins | **15–20** mins

200g rolled oats
200g mixed seeds
15 soft pitted dates, diced
125g butter (or coconut oil)
2 tbsp honey
1 tsp ground cinnamon

COOK'S TIP
The flapjacks will keep
in an airtight container
for up to 7 days.

When the kids were young, I made mounds of flapjacks, with gallons of golden syrup, which is essentially refined sugar with water. Yes, they were popular, but with a few simple tweaks, such as using diced dates instead of sugar and adding seeds for extra fibre and protein, they still wolfed them down. For reluctant seed eaters, just chop the larger seeds smaller before adding to the mixture.

1. Preheat the oven to 190°C/Fan 170°C/Gas 5 and line a 18cm square tin with non-stick baking paper.

2. Combine the oats and seeds in a medium mixing bowl.

3. Place 1 tablespoon of water in a small pan over a gentle heat. Add the diced dates, then use the back of a spoon to soften them and make a paste.

4. Add the butter or coconut oil, honey, cinnamon and a generous pinch of salt to the pan, then bring to a gentle simmer.

5. Stir the date mixture into the oats and seeds until coated. Press the mixture firmly into the prepared tin and bake in the oven for about 15–20 minutes.

6. Remove from the oven and leave to cool before cutting into 16 slices.

PER SERVING / 189 CALS / PROTEIN 4.7G / SUGAR 3.9G / FIBRE 2.3G / CARBS 13.1G

Vanilla Sesame Seed Biscuits

SERVES **12**

PREP **10** mins

COOK **12** mins

75g tahini
2 tbsp honey
1 medium free-range egg
1 tbsp vanilla extract
Zest of 1 lemon (optional)
150g ground almonds
½ tsp bicarbonate of soda
30g white sesame seeds
   (or a mix of white and black)

COOK'S TIP
Store the biscuits in
an airtight container.

A sophisticated and moreish nibble, and a wonderful treat to crumble over fruit puddings for extra texture and flavour. Sesame seeds are highly nutritious, providing healthy fats, fibre and antioxidants. They may even help reduce blood sugars and combat arthritis.

1. Preheat the oven to 190°C/Fan 170°C/Gas 5 and line two baking trays with non-stick baking paper.

2. Place the tahini, honey, egg, vanilla extract and lemon zest, if using, in a food processor or blender and blitz until combined.

3. Add the ground almonds, bicarbonate of soda and a pinch of sea salt and blitz again briefly.

4. Divide the mixture into 12 pieces and roll until smooth.

5. Tip the sesame seeds into a bowl, then roll each ball in the seeds until covered. Place the biscuits on the prepared baking trays and flatten them slightly with the back of a spoon. Bake in the oven for 12 minutes, or until golden brown and crisp around the edges.

6. Leave to cool on a wire rack.

PER SERVING / 154 CALS / PROTEIN 5.7G / SUGAR 3.6G / FIBRE 0.9G / CARBS 3.9G

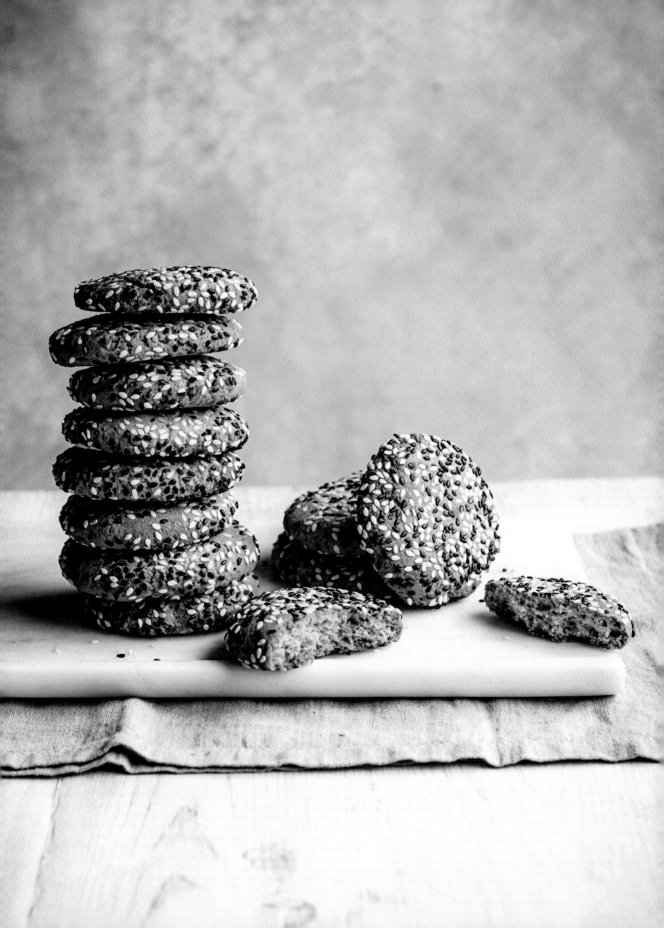

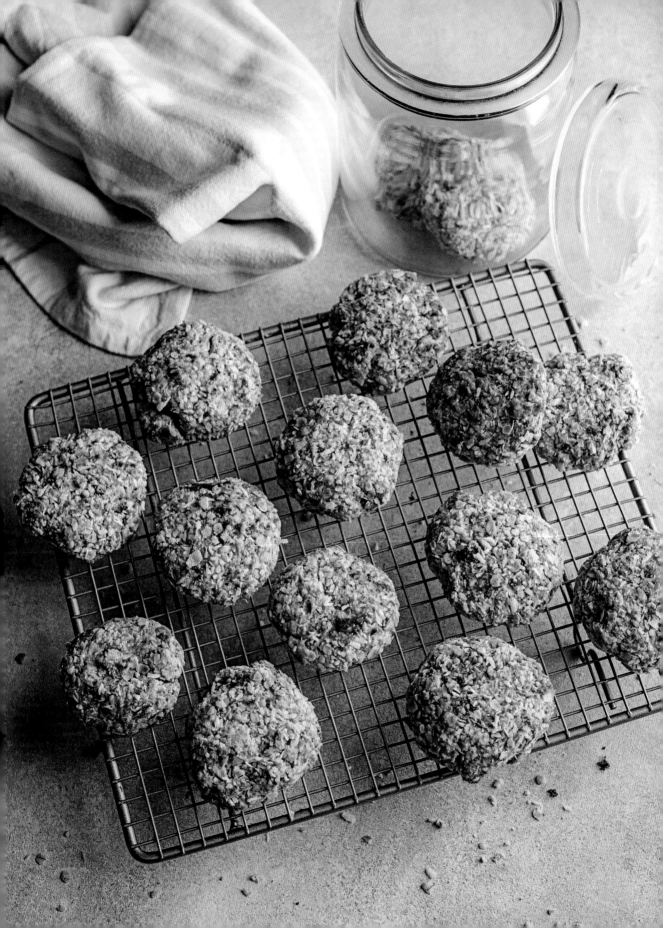

Coconut Anzac Biscuits

MAKES **16**

PREP **10** mins

COOK **15–20** mins

120g wholegrain spelt flour
90g rolled oats
100g desiccated coconut
1 tsp baking powder
185g soft pitted dates, diced
125g butter (or coconut oil)
1 tbsp honey

COOK'S TIP
Store the biscuits in
an airtight container.

My wonderful mother-in-law used to cook these classic coconut-flavoured biscuits; the recipe was passed on to her by her lovely sister in Australia. With a few small tweaks, I hope I do them justice. Spelt or buckwheat flours are higher in fibre than most other flours and should be available in most big supermarkets.

1. Preheat the oven to 190°C/Fan 170°C/Gas 5 and line a baking tray with non-stick baking paper.

2. Mix the spelt flour, oats, coconut and baking powder in a medium bowl along with a generous pinch of salt.

3. Place the diced dates in a small saucepan with 1 tablespoon of water and simmer gently for a few minutes, then use the back of a spoon to soften them into a paste. Add the butter or oil to the pan and stir in the honey. Turn off the heat and mix.

4. Add the date mixture to the dry ingredients and stir together well.

5. Divide the mixture into 16 walnut-sized pieces, then roll them into balls and place on the prepared baking tray. Flatten them slightly with the back of a spoon or your thumb and bake in the oven for 15–20 minutes until golden brown around the edges.

6. Leave to cool on a wire rack.

PER SERVING / 167 CALS / PROTEIN 2.2G / SUGAR 4.9G / FIBRE 2.6G / CARBS 13.7G

Apple and Peanut Butter 'Bagel'

SERVES
1

PREP
5
mins

1 medium apple, cored
1 tbsp unsweetened
    peanut butter
½ tsp ground cinnamon,
    or more to taste

For an instant, healthy treat, apples and peanut butter are a great-tasting combination. They are taken to another level here with the addition of cinnamon. This 'bagel' is a fun way to enjoy the pectin in apples, while also delivering prebiotic fibre to feed your gut microbes. It's become my new favourite instant snack!

1. Slice the cored apple around the middle into 3–4mm discs to produce 4–5 bagel-shaped slices.

2. Spread each slice with peanut butter, then sprinkle with the cinnamon to serve.

PER SERVING / 170 CALS / PROTEIN 4.8G / SUGAR 16.4G / FIBRE 2.7G / CARBS 18.8G

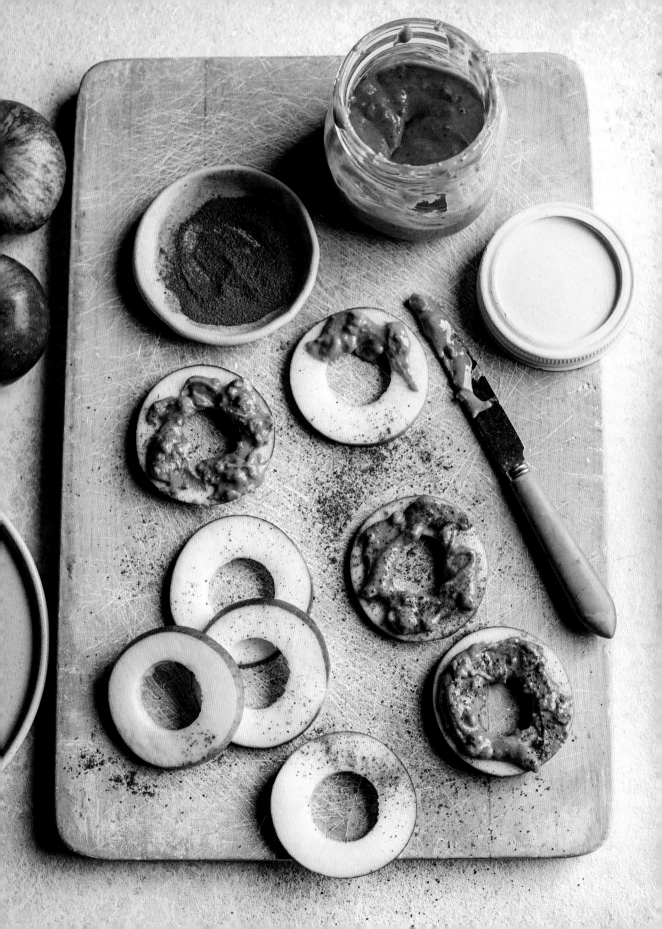

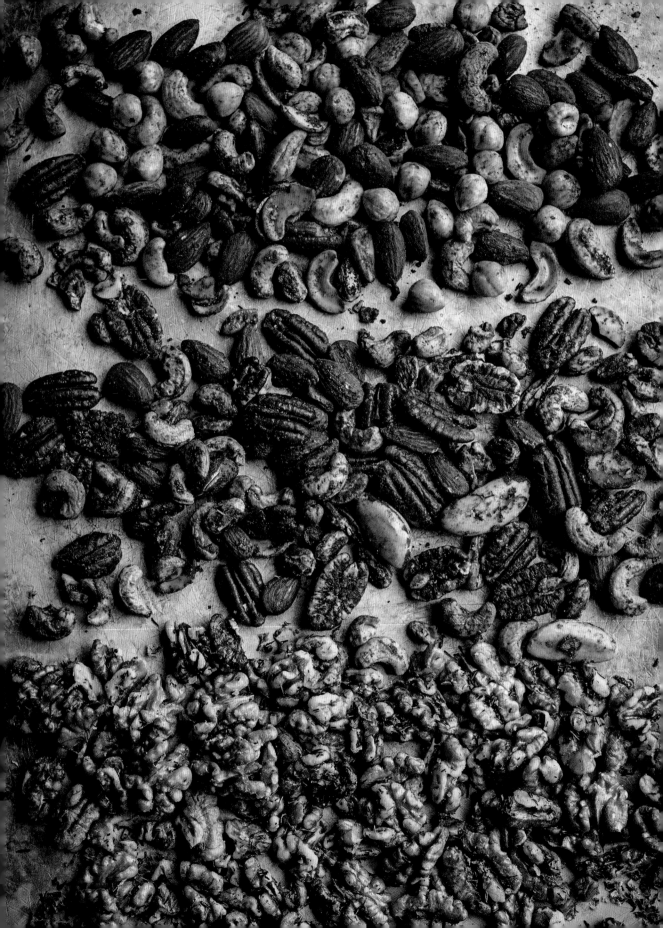

Savoury Trail Mix – Three Flavours

MAKES	PREP	COOK
200g	**5** mins	**7–10** mins

Whether you fancy paprika and chilli, Mediterranean thyme with lemon and sea salt, or the more exotic five spice and honey, these trail mixes make a flavoursome and satisfying snack. It's also a great way to use up half-empty bags of nuts that might be lurking in your cupboard. For ease, buy ready-mixed bags of nuts in the supermarket. Walnuts, almonds, Brazil nuts, hazelnuts and cashew nuts work particularly well. The amount of time to cook the nuts varies depending on size, so keep a close eye after they have been in the oven for 5 minutes, and check every 2 minutes after that.

VEGAN GLUTEN FREE DAIRY FREE

Paprika and Chilli

200g mixed nuts
1½ tsp paprika
½ tsp cayenne pepper
   (add 1 tsp if you like spice)
1 tbsp olive oil
½ tsp sea salt

1. Preheat the oven to 190°C/Fan 170°C/Gas 5. Line a baking tray with non-stick baking paper.

2. Mix all the ingredients together in a medium bowl, until the nuts are thoroughly coated in the spice.

3. Transfer the nuts to the prepared baking tray in a single layer, then roast in the oven for about 7 minutes until golden brown and fragrant. Allow to cool and serve immediately, or store in an airtight container for up to 1 week.

PER SERVING / 130 CALS / PROTEIN 5.5G / SUGAR 1.1G / FIBRE 0.1G / CARBS 2.2G

Walnuts with Thyme, Lemon and Sea Salt

200g walnuts
2 tsp dried thyme
Zest of 1 lemon
1½ tbsp olive oil
½ tsp sea salt

1. Preheat the oven to 190°C/Fan 170°C/Gas 5. Line a baking tray with non-stick baking paper.

2. Mix all the ingredients together in a medium bowl, until the nuts are thoroughly coated in the lemon and herbs.

3. Transfer the nuts to the prepared baking tray in a single layer, then roast for 7–10 minutes, or until deep golden and crispy. Allow to cool and serve immediately, or store in an airtight container for up to 1 week.

PER SERVING / 156 CALS / PROTEIN 3.5G / SUGAR 0.5G / FIBRE 0.9G / CARBS 0.6G

Chinese Five Spice and Honey

200g mixed nuts
1 tsp honey
1 tsp Chinese five spice powder
1 tsp olive oil
½ tsp sea salt

1. Preheat the oven to 190°C/Fan 170°C/Gas 5. Line a baking tray with non-stick baking paper.

2. Mix all the ingredients together in a medium bowl, until the nuts are thoroughly coated in the honey and spice.

3. Transfer to the prepared baking tray in a single layer, then roast in the oven for about 7 minutes until golden brown and fragrant. Allow to cool and serve immediately, or store in an airtight container for up to 1 week.

PER SERVING / 124 CALS / PROTEIN 5.5G / SUGAR 1.6G / FIBRE 0.1G / CARBS 2.8G

Chocolate Pennies – Three Ways

MAKES | **PREP** | **SET**
20 | **15** mins | **2–3** hours

100g dark chocolate
(at least 70%)

Topping One
20g toasted flaked almonds,
roughly chopped
5g freeze-dried raspberries,
roughly chopped

Topping Two
½ tsp cayenne pepper
20g dried mango,
finely chopped

Topping Three
2 tbsp desiccated coconut

COOK'S TIP
If you can't find ready-toasted almonds, sprinkle plain flaked almonds into a small frying pan and toast over a medium heat for 3–4 minutes, stirring regularly. Don't leave them unattended as they can quickly burn. Leave to cool before sprinkling over the melted chocolate.

These small, elegant dark chocolate coins are rich in beneficial polyphenols, which are potent antioxidants, reducing inflammation in the body. And your gut microbiome will love them, too. Choose your favourite topping, or mix and match. The quantities of toppings are for one set of 20 coins.

1. Line a large baking tray with non-stick baking paper.

2. Place the chocolate in a microwave-safe bowl and microwave for 30 seconds, then in bursts of 15 seconds (so as not to overheat it or the chocolate will stiffen and burn), until melted.

3. Using a teaspoon, pour 20 individual spoonfuls of the melted chocolate on to the prepared baking tray, spaced well apart.

4. Scatter your chosen topping on top of the melted chocolate. Leave to set for 2–3 hours.

5. Place in an airtight container and store for up to a week in a cool place (best not to store in the fridge as the chocolate could discolour).

PER SERVING / 40 CALS / PROTEIN 0.5G / SUGAR 4G / FIBRE 0G / CARBS 4.2G

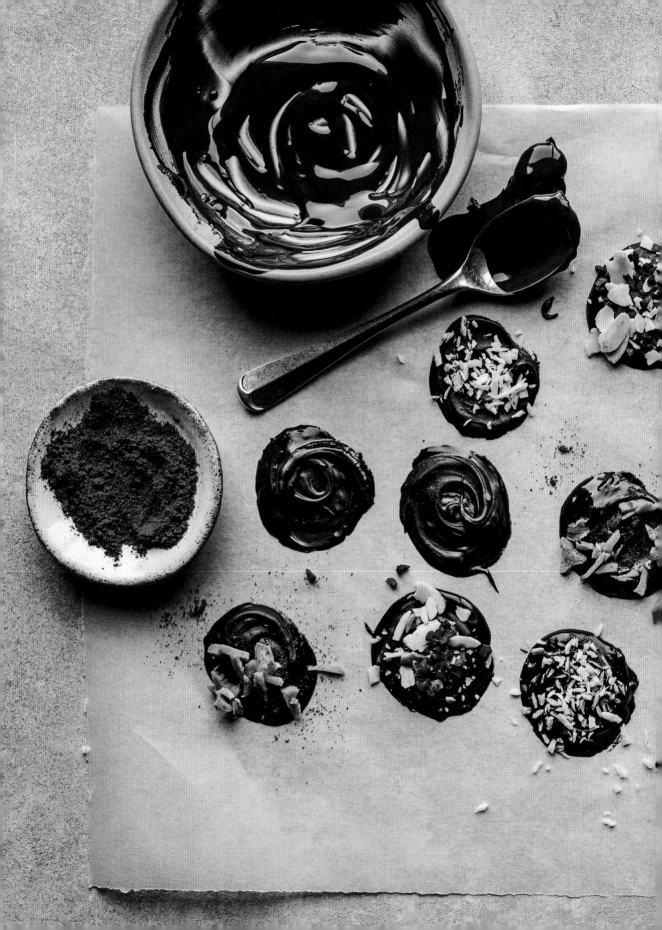

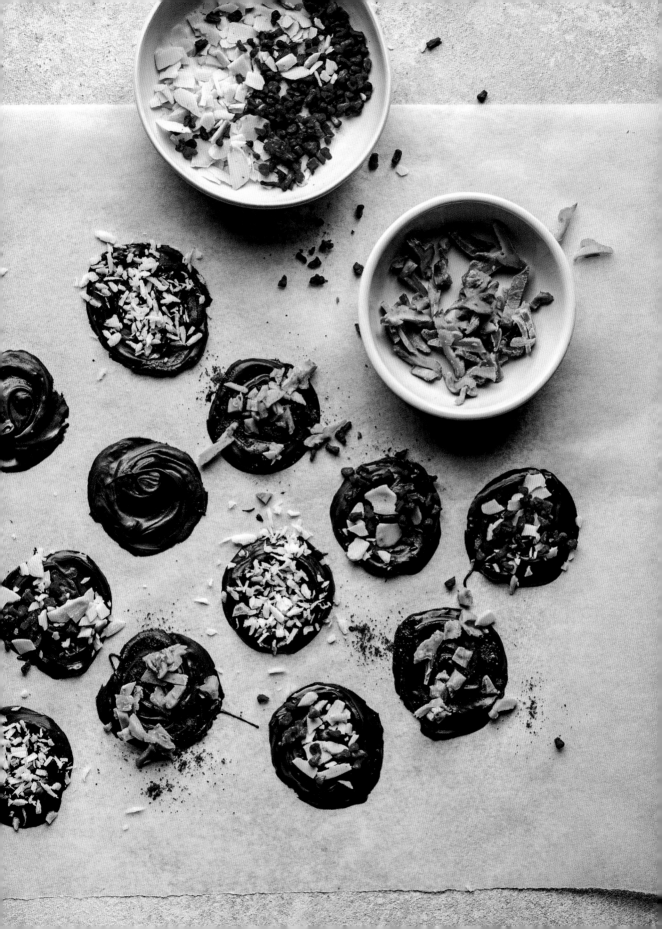

Nutty Chocolate Orange Fridge Brownies

MAKES
9

PREP
15
mins

SET
2
hours

100g pecan nuts
100g ground almonds
50g unsweetened
   cocoa powder
100g soft pitted dates
4 tbsp coconut oil
1 large ripe banana
   (or 2 small), peeled
   and mashed
Zest of 1 orange

COOK'S TIP
Along with the orange zest, scatter some extra pecan nuts on top of the brownies and press them firmly into the mixture for decoration if you wish.

These brownies will keep in the fridge for 3–4 days.

Sweetened by fruit and packed with fibre and protein, these super-healthy, orange-flavoured bars might become a favourite. They are ideal in a lunch box, good enjoyed with a coffee or great as a dessert with a spoonful of Greek yoghurt. And you don't even need to turn the oven on.

1. Line a 18cm square tin with non-stick baking paper.

2. Place the pecan nuts, ground almonds, cocoa powder, dates, coconut oil, mashed banana and three quarters of the orange zest in the bowl of an electric mixer, and whiz until smooth but retaining a bit of texture.

3. Transfer the mixture to the prepared tin and flatten with a spatula until tightly packed.

4. Scatter the remaining orange zest over the surface of the brownies, then refrigerate for at least 2 hours before cutting into 9 squares.

PER SERVING / 283 CALS / PROTEIN 6.2G / SUGAR 11.1G / FIBRE 2.6G / CARBS 12.6G

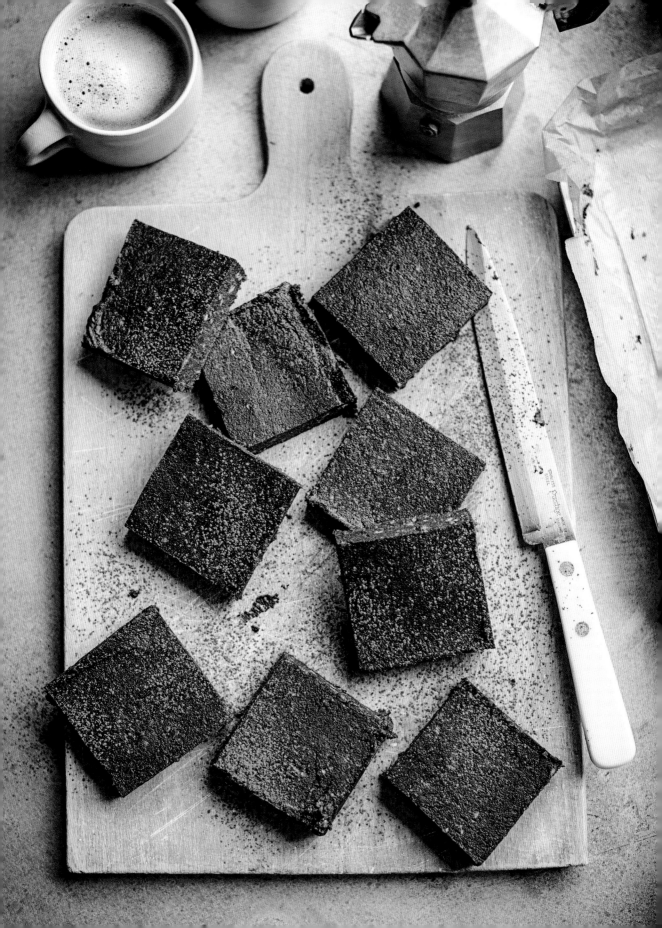

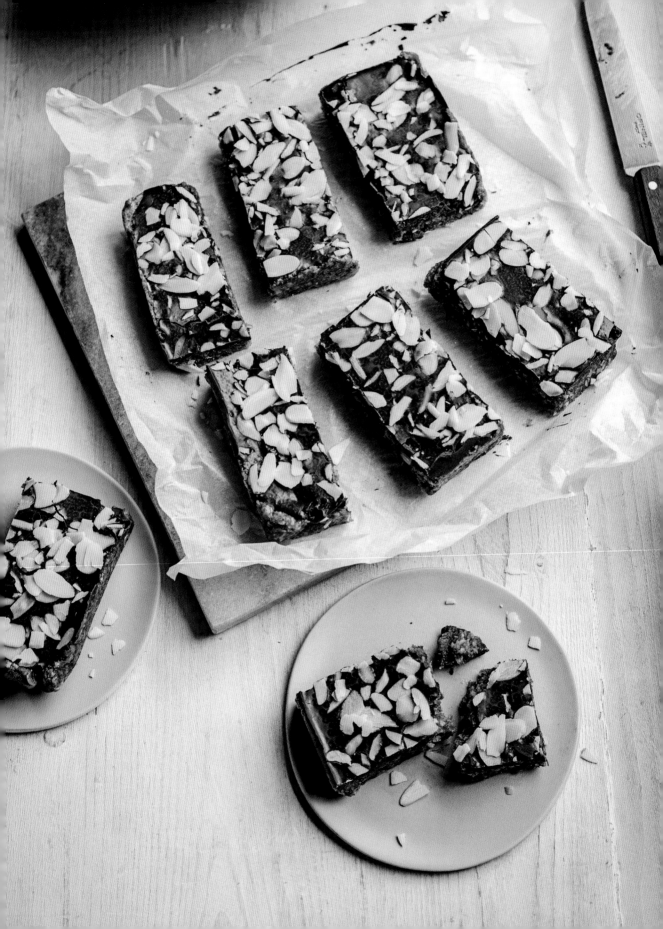

Chocolate Almond Fridge Bars

MAKES | **PREP** | **SET**
8 | **15** mins | **1–2** hours

135g almond butter
1 tbsp honey
100g rolled oats
9 soft pitted dates
90g dark chocolate
(at least 70%)
10g flaked almonds

COOK'S TIP
These will keep in
the fridge for 3–4 days.

Fridge bars are so easy to blitz together and require no baking. These enticing snacks are a winner that shouldn't give a sugar spike, especially if enjoyed after a meal.

1. Line a 18cm square tin with non-stick baking paper.

2. Place the almond butter, honey, oats, dates and 2 tablespoons of water in an electric mixer and blitz until the mixture resembles wet breadcrumbs.

3. Transfer to the prepared tin and press down firmly until the mixture is tightly packed and smooth on the surface.

4. Place the chocolate in a microwave-safe bowl and heat for 30 seconds, then in bursts of 15 seconds, stirring each time, until melted.

5. Pour the chocolate over the almond base, spread out evenly, then scatter the flaked almonds on top. Refrigerate for 1–2 hours, until set, then slice into 8 bars.

PER SERVING / 246 CALS / PROTEIN 5.9G / SUGAR 15.9G / FIBRE 2G / CARBS 34.7G

Chocolate Cherry Coconut Bars

MAKES
6

PREP
20 mins

SET
1 hour

100g desiccated coconut
160ml coconut cream
1 tsp vanilla paste (or 2 tbsp vanilla extract)
100g tinned cherries, drained
150g dark chocolate (at least 70%), broken into pieces

COOK'S TIP
If you prefer not to coat the bars fully, you could use less chocolate and only pour a thick layer on the top. Store in the fridge for up to 5 days or keep in the freezer.

I do love the occasional chocolate coconut bar, so I'm delighted to have created a surprisingly luxurious healthy version with the addition of cherries to the filling.

1. Line a 900g loaf tin with non-stick baking paper or tin foil, allowing an overhang so you can easily lift out the contents.

2. Mix the desiccated coconut, coconut cream, vanilla, cherries and a pinch of salt in a medium bowl. Blitz briefly with a hand-held blender to combine.

3. Press the mixture into the base of the prepared tin and transfer to the freezer for about 1 hour to set.

4. Place the chocolate in a microwave-safe bowl and microwave for 30 seconds, then in bursts of 15 seconds, stirring each time, until melted.

5. Remove the tin from the freezer and lift out the coconut loaf. Cut into 6 bars, separating them from each other using a knife. Pour some chocolate over the top of each one, spreading it out to cover. Transfer the bars to a plate and pop in the fridge for 1–2 minutes to set the chocolate.

6. Remove the plate from the fridge, turn the bars over and pour more chocolate on another side. Repeat until they are completely covered.

PER SERVING / 313 CALS / PROTEIN 3.1G / SUGAR 19.5G / FIBRE 4G / CARBS 21.6G

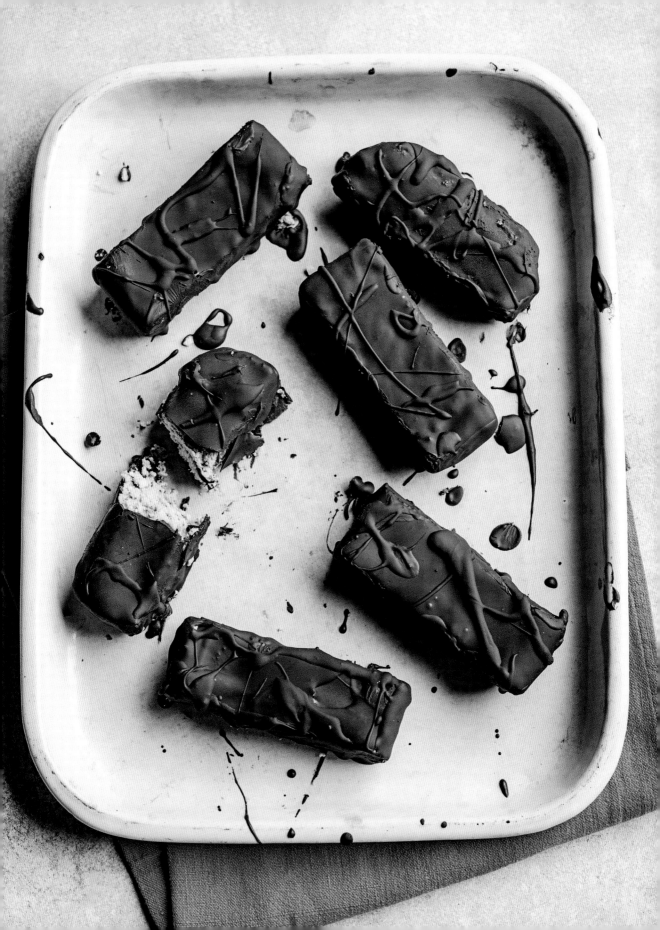

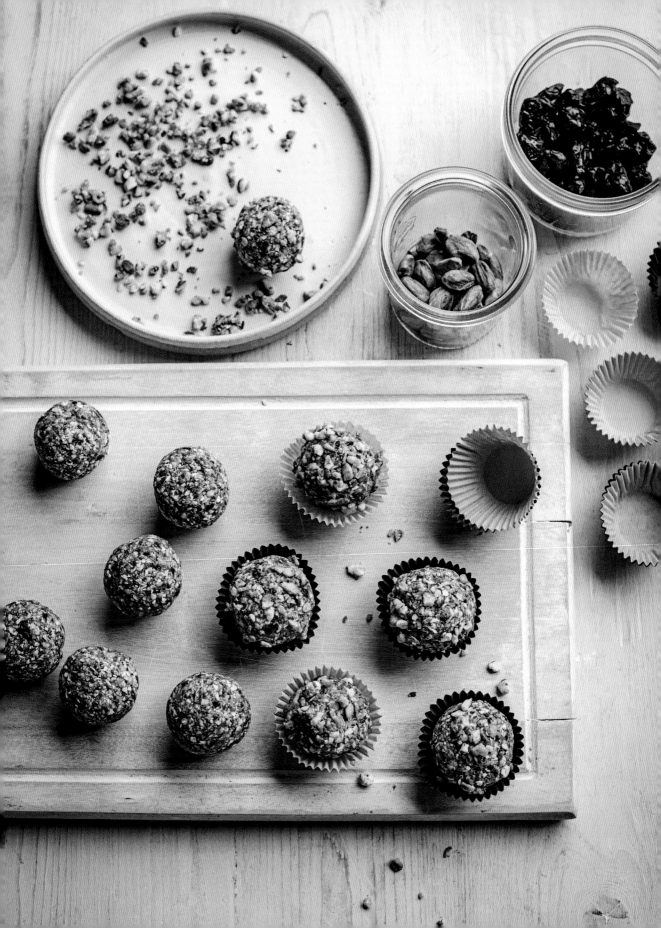

Pistachio and Cranberry Bliss Balls

MAKES
12

PREP
15
mins

80g soft pitted dates
1 tbsp chia seeds
1 tbsp honey
1 tbsp tahini
80g jumbo oats
80g shelled pistachios
35g dried cranberries

COOK'S TIP
Store in the fridge
and eat within 1 week.

Bursting with fruit, protein and healthy nutrients, these bliss balls are a perfect snack. They fill that little gap after a meal, are ideal packed in a lunch box or eaten after a work-out to boost your energy. Just blitz and roll them together!

1. Place the dates, chia seeds, honey and tahini in a food processor or blender and blitz until smooth. Use a spatula to scrape down the sides.

2. Add the oats, 60g of the pistachios, the dried cranberries, a pinch of salt and 2 tablespoons of water. Blitz until the mixture is finely chopped and starting to clump together. Squeeze some of the mixture between your fingers – if it sticks together easily it is ready. If not, add another tablespoon of water and blitz again.

3. Divide the mixture into 12 and roll each piece tightly between the palms of your hands into a ball.

4. Finely chop the remaining pistachios, then tip this into a bowl. Roll each bliss ball in the chopped nuts.

PER SERVING / 109 CALS / PROTEIN 2.9G / SUGAR 7.4G / FIBRE 1.7G / CARBS 12.8G

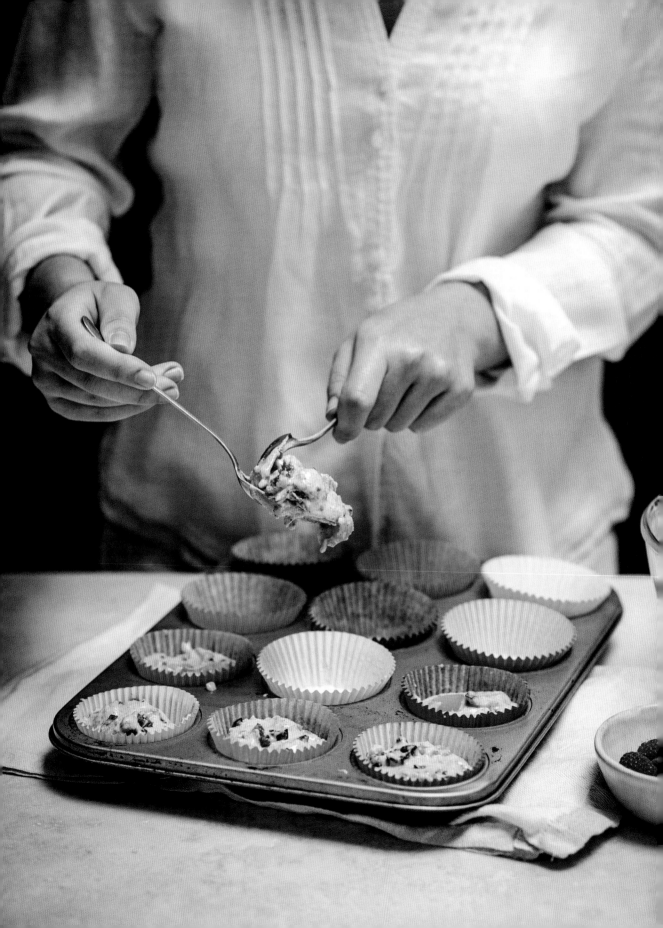

Cupcakes & Muffins

Raspberry, Peach and Chocolate Cupcakes

MAKES **12** | **PREP** **15** mins | **COOK** **15** mins

1 × 150ml pot of natural full-fat yoghurt, or dairy-free equivalent

1 pot olive oil (150ml)

1 pot peaches drained from a tin (ideally stored in fruit juice), finely diced (85g)

1 pot dark chocolate chunks (at least 70%) (85g)

2 tsp baking powder

3 medium free-range eggs

1 pot ground almonds (70g)

1 pot wholegrain buckwheat flour (100g)

1 tbsp honey

1 pot fresh or frozen raspberries (75g)

This is a favourite in the Mosley household. The ingredients can be measured using the yoghurt pot, so there's no fiddling with scales – perfect for cooking with kids. If you don't have a small yoghurt pot, use a generous ½ cup measure (about 125–150ml).

1. Preheat the oven to 190°C/Fan 170°C/Gas 5. Line a 12-hole cupcake tin with paper cases.

2. Place all the ingredients, except the raspberries, in a bowl with a pinch of salt and mix thoroughly.

3. Gently stir in half of the raspberries, then divide the mixture between the paper cases. Top the cupcakes with the remaining raspberries and bake in the oven for 15 minutes, or until golden brown and a skewer inserted into the centre comes out clean.

4. Leave to cool on a wire rack.

———

PER SERVING / 229 CALS / PROTEIN 5.3G / SUGAR 7.8G / FIBRE 0.8G / CARBS 15G

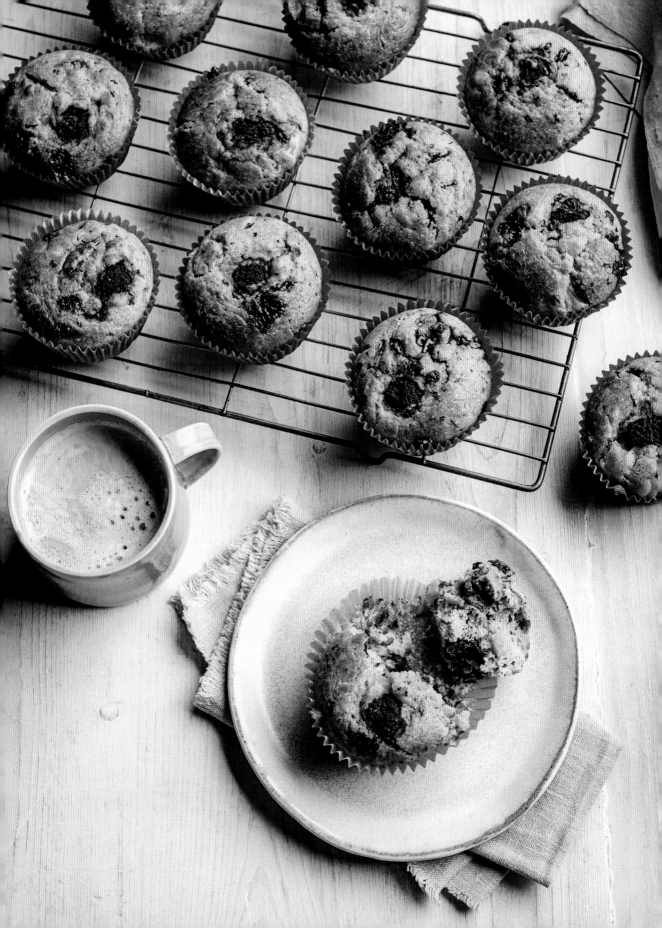

Double Dark Chocolate Cupcakes

MAKES	PREP	COOK
8	**10** mins	**15–20** mins

150g ground almonds

2½ tbsp unsweetened
cocoa powder

1 tbsp baking powder

1 tbsp vanilla extract

1 large ripe banana
(or 2 small), peeled
and broken into chunks

2 medium free-range eggs

1 tbsp honey (optional)

50g coconut oil, melted

75g dark chocolate buttons

For the Icing

80g mascarpone cheese,
or dairy-free equivalent

1 tsp honey

15g dark chocolate
(at least 70%), finely grated

Double dark chocolate indulgence. You might be surprised to hear that not only is cocoa one of the richest sources of health-enhancing polyphenols, it is also as much as 30% fibre, so your gut microbiome benefits when you eat it, too. What's more, cocoa has been shown to reduce inflammation, improve blood pressure and reduce blood sugars.

1. Preheat the oven to 190°C/Fan 170°C/Gas 5. Line a 12-hole cupcake tin with 8 paper cases.

2. Place the ground almonds, cocoa powder, baking powder, vanilla extract, banana, eggs, honey, if using, and a pinch of salt in a food processor or blender and blitz until you have a smooth batter. Add the coconut oil and blitz again.

3. Fold the chocolate buttons into the batter, then divide the mixture between the paper cases. Bake in the oven for 15–20 minutes, or until a skewer inserted into the centre comes out clean. Leave to cool on a wire rack.

4. Meanwhile, mix the mascarpone, honey and most of the grated chocolate together in a small bowl to make the icing.

5. Spread the icing on to the cooled cupcakes, then sprinkle over the remaining grated chocolate to serve.

PER SERVING / 336 CALS / PROTEIN 9.3G / SUGAR 11.2G / FIBRE 1.3G / CARBS 13.2G

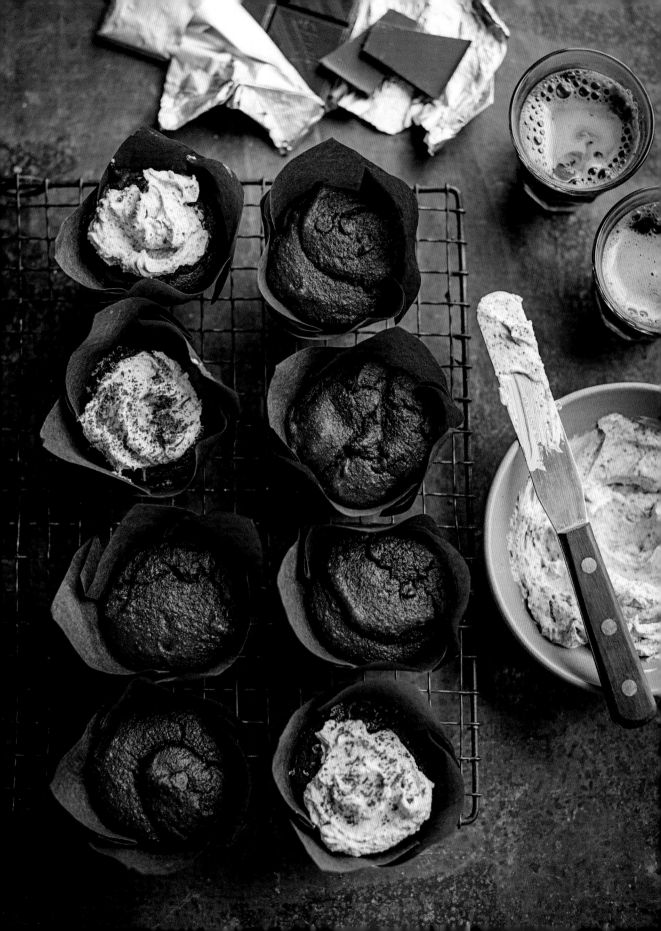

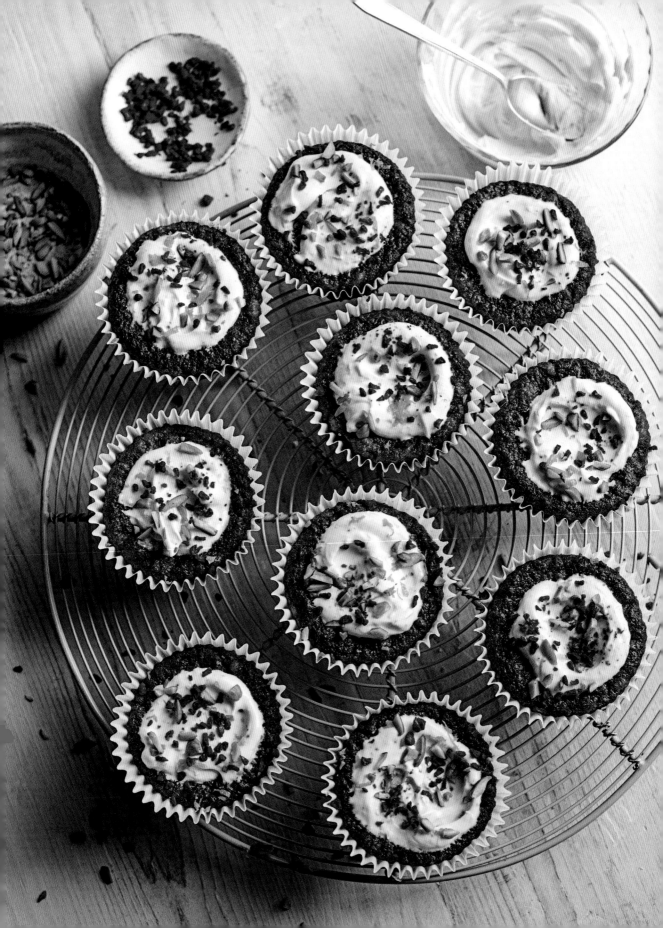

Iced Apricot and Orange Cupcakes

MAKES | **PREP** | **COOK**
12 | **15** mins | **18–20** mins

100g dried apricots,
   finely chopped
60g coconut oil
   (or butter) melted
2 medium free-range eggs
60g shelled pistachios,
   roughly chopped
Zest and juice of
   2 medium oranges
100g ground almonds
1 tsp ground cinnamon
1 tsp ground cardamom
   (optional)
1 tsp bicarbonate of soda
2 tbsp freeze-dried raspberries
1 tbsp cider vinegar

For the Icing
120g full-fat cream cheese,
   or dairy-free equivalent
1½ tsp honey
1 tsp lemon zest

COOK'S TIP
The cupcakes freeze
well uniced.

Loosely based on a Persian love cake, these enchantingly rich and exotic cupcakes have a tangy, orange-flavoured topping and a rich, nutty base. With such delicious and healthy ingredients, you can't really go wrong. This is a fairly heavy, flavourful cake – don't expect a light fluffy sponge – but is one of my favourites.

1. Preheat the oven to 190°C/Fan 170°C/Gas 5. Line a 12-hole cupcake tin with paper cases.

2. Place the apricots, coconut oil or butter and eggs in a bowl and blitz with a hand-held blender for about 30 seconds, or until creamy but retaining some texture.

3. Stir in 40g of the pistachios, all the orange juice, half the orange zest, the ground almonds, cinnamon, cardamom, if using, bicarbonate of soda, half the dried raspberries and a generous pinch of salt. Mix well, then add the cider vinegar and mix again.

4. Divide the mixture between the paper cases and bake for 18–20 minutes, or until golden brown and a skewer inserted into the centre comes out clean. Leave to cool on a wire rack.

5. Meanwhile, mix the remaining orange zest with the cream cheese, honey and lemon zest in a small bowl to make the icing. Spread this on to the cooled cupcakes, then sprinkle the remaining chopped pistachios and dried raspberries on top.

PER SERVING / 189 CALS / PROTEIN 5.4G / SUGAR 6.4G / FIBRE 0.9G / CARBS 7.6G

Cherry and Pistachio Buckwheat Cupcakes

MAKES **12**

PREP **10** mins

COOK **15–20** mins

150g tinned cherries, drained
50g butter, softened
125ml full-fat milk
60g full-fat Greek yoghurt
1 medium free-range egg
1 tbsp vanilla extract
1½ tbsp maple syrup
1 medium very ripe
   banana, peeled
150g wholegrain
   buckwheat flour
1 tsp baking powder
¾ tsp bicarbonate of soda
30g shelled pistachios,
   roughly chopped

Although fresh cherries when they are out of season are a bit of a luxury, tinned cherries are easily available, deliciously sweet and are an excellent healthy alternative. In fact, frozen and tinned foods are often fresher than their 'fresh' counterparts. Some of the benefits of cherries include reducing blood pressure, blood sugars and inflammatory conditions. They may even improve sleep.

1. Preheat the oven to 190°C/Fan 170°C/Gas 5 and line a 12-hole cupcake tin with paper cases.

2. Place the drained cherries between two pieces of kitchen roll and squeeze out the excess liquid. Roughly chop and set aside.

3. Place the butter, milk, yoghurt, egg, vanilla extract, maple syrup and banana in a medium bowl and use a hand-held blender to blitz until smooth.

4. Add the buckwheat flour, baking powder and bicarbonate of soda and stir until combined.

5. Fold in the cherries and pistachios and divide between the paper cases. Bake in the oven for 15–20 minutes, or until golden brown and a skewer inserted in the centre comes out clean.

PER SERVING / 133 CALS / PROTEIN 3.2G / SUGAR 5.9G / FIBRE 0.6G / CARBS 16.5G

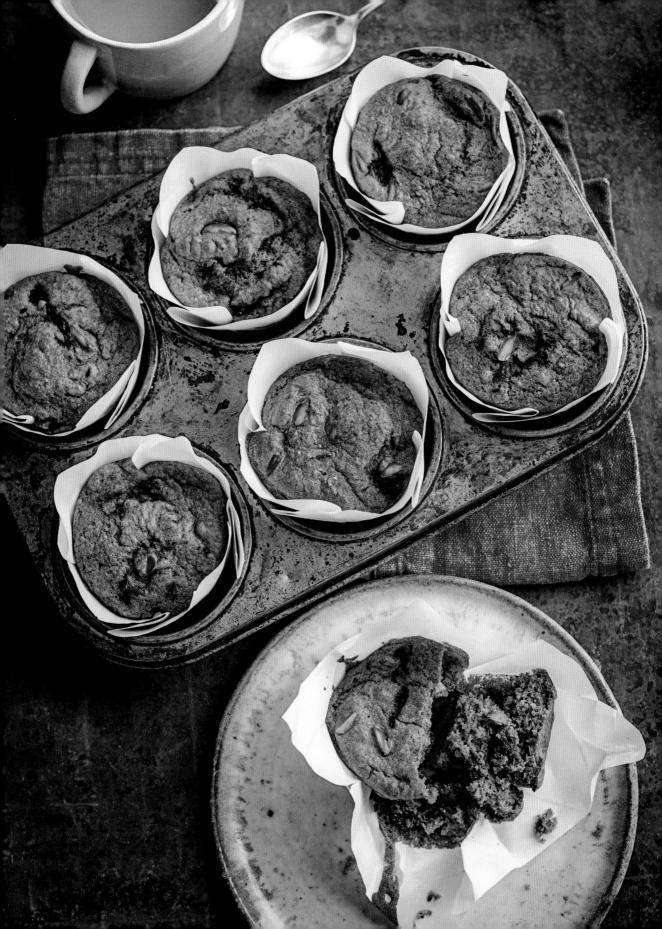

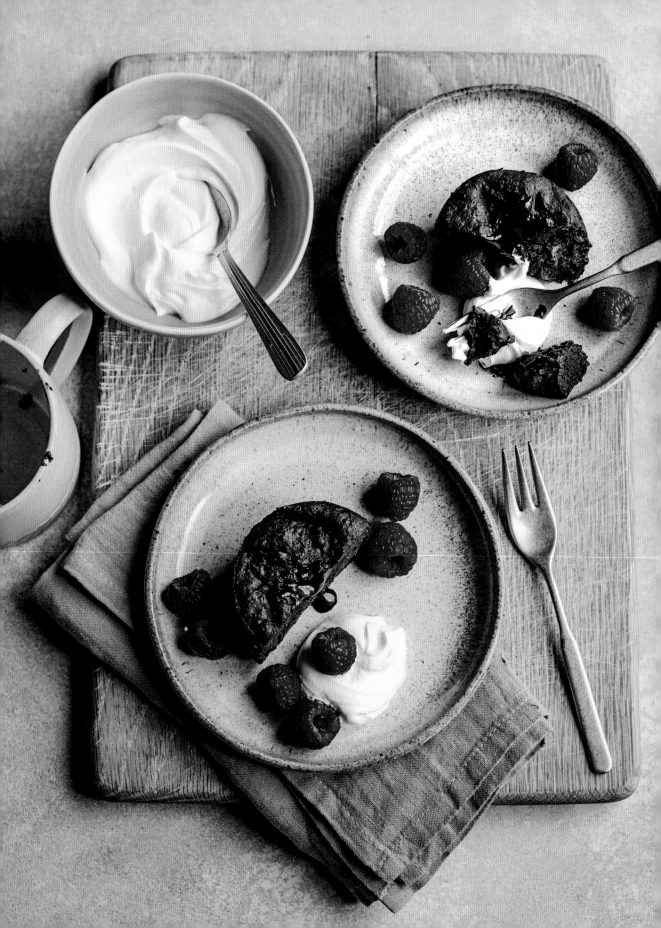

All-time-favourite Chocolate Mug Cake

SERVES **2** | **PREP** **5** mins | **COOK** **2** mins

1 tbsp coconut oil
1 medium free-range egg,
    beaten well
4 soft pitted dates,
    finely chopped
25g ground almonds
1 tbsp unsweetened
    cocoa powder
¼ tsp baking powder
1 square dark chocolate
    (at least 70%) (around 5g)
Handful of fresh raspberries,
    to serve (optional)

COOK'S TIP
This would also go well
with a dollop of Greek
or dairy-free yoghurt.

Unbelievably instant gooey-centred chocolate indulgence. Made in minutes, this is so easy to cook, anyone could do it, including kids. My young nephew loves making this.

1. Place the coconut oil in a microwave-proof mug (to hold around 300ml) and melt in the microwave on high for a few seconds. Do not allow to overheat. Use a spatula to spread the oil all around the inside of the mug.

2. Add the egg, dates, ground almonds, cocoa powder and baking powder and, using a fork, mix the ingredients until thoroughly combined.

3. Press the square of chocolate into the top of the cake batter and place the mug in the microwave. Cook on high for about 1½ minutes, or until the cake is risen, firm and just beginning to shrink from the sides of the mug.

4. Holding the hot mug carefully, turn the cake out on to a plate and cut in half to reveal the melted chocolate.

5. Divide between two plates and serve each half topped with a handful of fresh raspberries, if liked.

———

PER SERVING / 215 CALS / PROTEIN 8.2G / SUGAR 6.5G / FIBRE 1G / CARBS 7.4G

Rhubarb and Cherry Mug Cake

SERVES	PREP	COOK
2	**5** mins	**2–3** mins

1 tbsp coconut oil

50g rhubarb, finely diced

1 tsp stem ginger syrup
  (from the jar)

4 tbsp ground almonds

¼ tsp baking powder

2 tsp vanilla extract

1 medium free-range egg

2 balls of stem ginger in syrup,
  drained and finely chopped

5 cherries from a tin, drained
  and finely chopped (or use
  fresh cherries if in season)

2 tbsp full-fat Greek yoghurt,
  or a dairy-free equivalent,
  to serve

Another luscious, instant microwaved indulgence. Perfect for an impatient cook! Ready in about 5 minutes.

1. Place the coconut oil in a microwave-proof mug (to hold around 300ml) and melt in the microwave on high for a few seconds. Do not allow to overheat. Use a spatula to spread the oil all around the inside of the mug.

2. Add the diced rhubarb and ginger syrup to the mug and microwave for 1 minute. Leave to cool a little, then add the ground almonds, baking powder, vanilla extract, egg, stem ginger and a pinch of salt. Mix everything together until thoroughly combined, then fold in the cherries.

3. Microwave on high for about 1½ minutes, or until the cake is risen, firm and just beginning to shrink from the sides of the mug.

4. Holding the hot mug carefully, turn the cake out on to a plate and cut in half.

5. Divide between two plates and serve each half topped with full-fat Greek yoghurt, or a dairy-free equivalent.

———

PER SERVING / 358 CALS / PROTEIN 12.7G / SUGAR 14.4G / FIBRE 0.8G / CARBS 17.1G

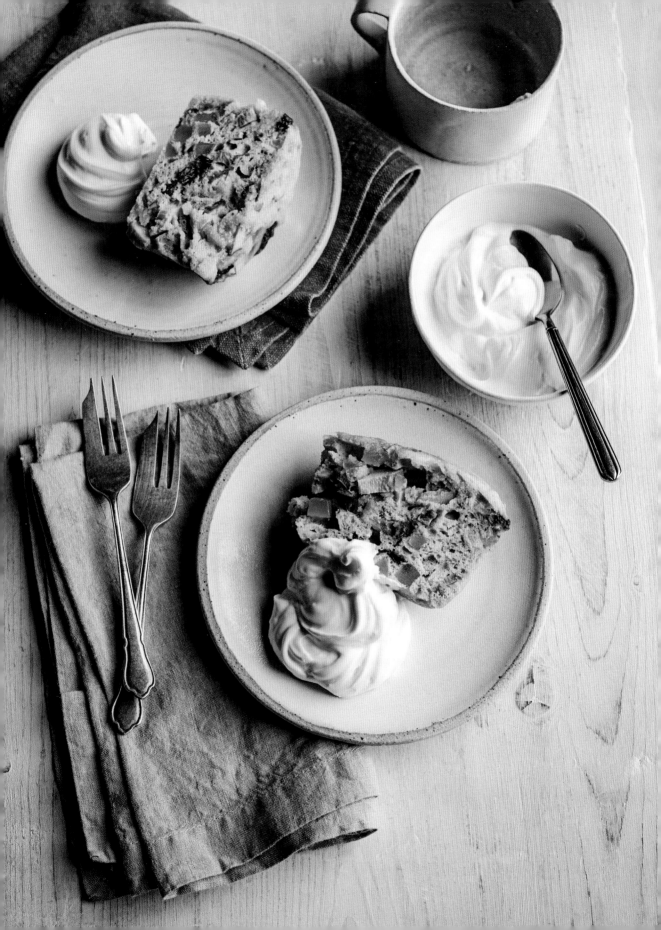

High-fibre Carrot and Pecan Muffins

MAKES | **PREP** | **COOK**
6 | **15** mins | **20–30** mins

50g pecan nuts (or walnuts)
1 large ripe banana (or 2 small),
    peeled and mashed
50g ground almonds
50g ground flax seeds
½ tbsp chia seeds (optional)
1 medium carrot, grated
3 tbsp full-fat Greek yoghurt,
    or dairy-free equivalent
40g dried cranberries, chopped
1 large or 2 small
    free-range eggs
2 tsp ground cinnamon
1 tsp bicarbonate of soda
1 tbsp honey

Perfect for boosting your gut microbiome, as well as keeping yourself 'regular', thanks to the wholesome high-fibre ingredients. But these are also delicious muffins and great for all the family. Naturally sweetened by ripe banana and a little honey, they are incredibly simple to make. Given that most of us don't get nearly enough fibre in our diets – here's a delicious way to top it up.

1. Preheat the oven to 180°C/Fan 160°C/Gas 4. Line a 12-hole muffin tin with 6 large silicone or paper cases.

2. Set aside 6 of the pecan nuts or walnuts, then roughly chop the rest.

3. Place the chopped nuts and all the remaining ingredients in a medium bowl with a pinch of salt and mix together well with an electric whisk.

4. Divide the mixture between the muffin cases, then press a whole pecan or walnut on to the top of each muffin. Bake for 20–30 minutes, or until a skewer inserted into the centre comes out clean.

5. Serve immediately or store in the fridge for up to 3 days.

PER SERVING / 234 CALS / PROTEIN 7.5G / SUGAR 13.3G / FIBRE 3.5G / CARBS 14.6G

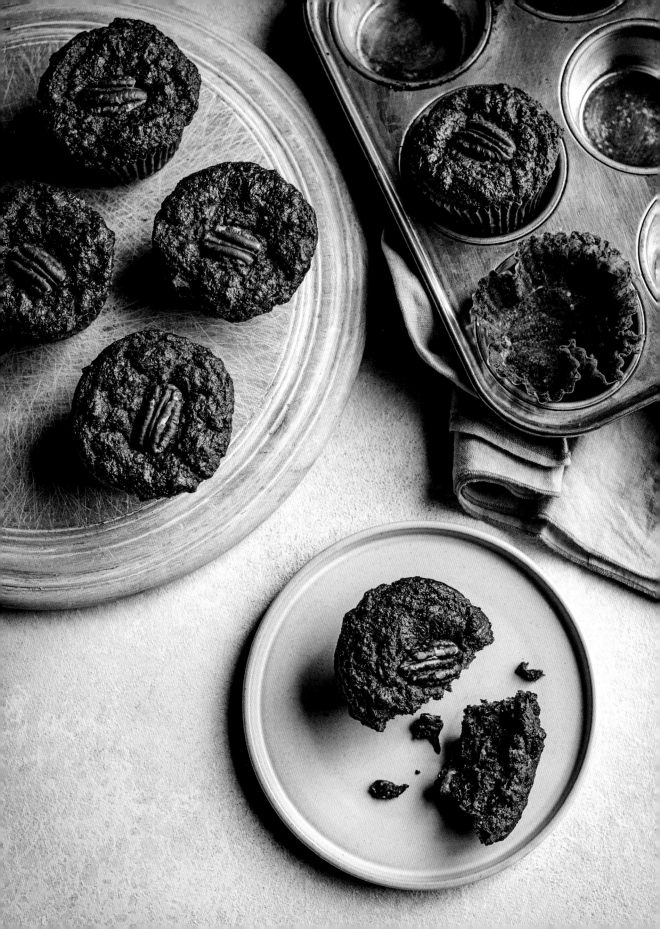

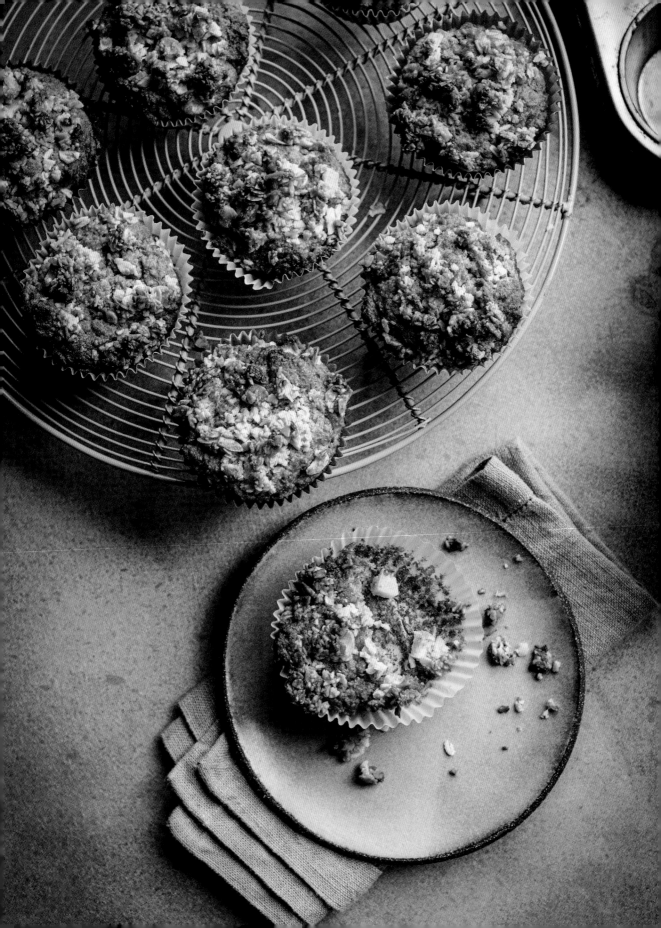

Apple and Banana Muffins with a Crumble Topping

MAKES **9** | **PREP** **20** mins | **COOK** **25** mins

1 medium eating apple, cored and finely diced, skin on
1 tbsp lemon juice
1½ tsp ground cinnamon
2 medium free-range eggs
1 medium ripe banana, peeled mashed
75g butter, softened
100g ground almonds
30g wholegrain spelt flour (or other wholegrain flour)
50g soft pitted dates, roughly chopped
1 tbsp vanilla extract
1½ tsp baking powder

For the Crumble Topping
50g flaked almonds
25g butter, softened
1 tsp maple syrup

Originally inspired by a tangy Dorset apple cake, we swapped the white flour for spelt flour, an ancient grain, which is higher in protein and fibre, and available in most major supermarkets.

1. Preheat the oven to 190°C/Fan 170°C/Gas 5. Line a 12-hole muffin tin with 9 paper cases.

2. To make the crumble topping, place the flaked almonds, butter and maple syrup in a small food processor or blender and blitz until you have a rough crumbly mixture. Set aside.

3. Place the diced apple in a medium bowl and toss with the lemon juice and cinnamon.

4. In a separate bowl, mix the eggs, banana, butter, ground almonds, flour, dates, vanilla extract and baking powder. Blitz with a hand-held blender to make a batter. Add the apple mixture and stir to combine.

5. Divide the batter between the muffin cases, top each one with a teaspoon of crumble and gently press it into the surface. Bake in the oven for 25 minutes, or until a skewer inserted into the centre comes out clean.

6. Leave to cool on a wire rack.

PER SERVING / 255 CALS / PROTEIN 6.9G / SUGAR 8.5G / FIBRE 1G / CARBS 11.7G

Throw-it-all-together Blueberry and Ginger Muffins

MAKES
8

PREP
10
mins

COOK
25
mins

50g butter, softened
  (or coconut oil, melted)
100g ground almonds
2 medium free-range eggs
3 balls of stem ginger in syrup,
  drained and finely chopped
2 tsp vanilla extract
1 tsp baking powder
150g blueberries

An easy 'chuck it all in and stir it together' muffin which is dark with delicious blueberries. Juicy and satisfying. Easy for kids to assemble.

1. Preheat the oven to 190°C/Fan 170°C/Gas 5. Line a 12-hole muffin tin with 8 paper cases.

2. Tip all the ingredients, except the blueberries, into a medium bowl and add a pinch of salt. Blitz the mixture using a hand-held blender or electric whisk until just combined. Fold in the blueberries.

3. Divide the mixture between the paper cases and bake in the oven for 25 minutes until golden brown.

4. Serve immediately or store in the fridge for up to 3 days.

PER SERVING / 213 CALS / PROTEIN 7.1G / SUGAR 4.4G / FIBRE 0.4G / CARBS 5.3G

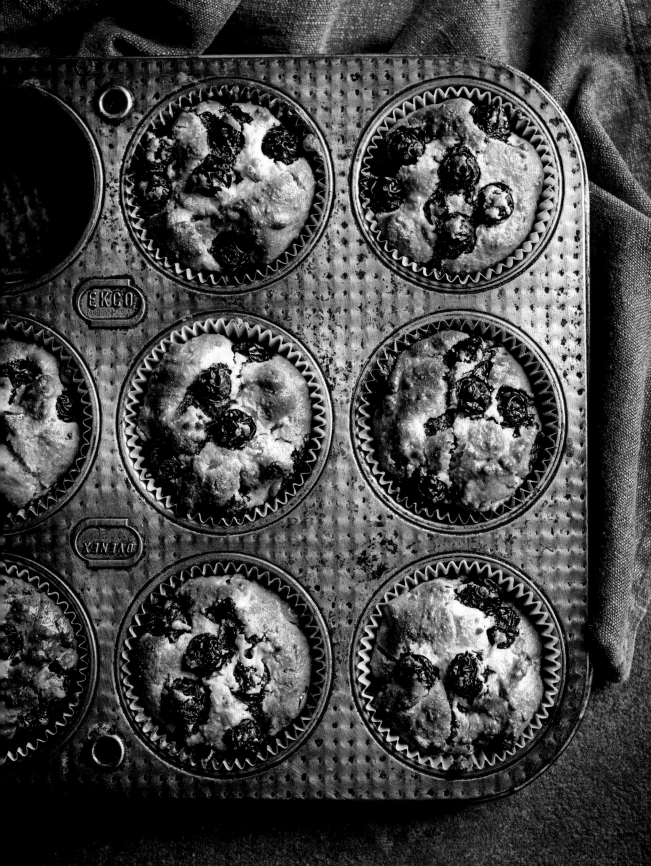

Basil and Feta Muffins with Pumpkin Seeds

MAKES | **PREP** | **COOK**
12 | **15** mins | **25** mins

1 large courgette (zucchini) (about 250g), trimmed and coarsely grated
150g ricotta
5 medium free-range eggs
180g wholegrain spelt flour
1 tsp baking powder
1 tsp salt
50g feta cheese, crumbled
50g pumpkin seeds
20g basil, leaves picked and finely chopped

High in protein and bursting with flavour, these really are a fabulous savoury treat. What's more, they are versatile, too, making an easy-to-grab breakfast, a satisfying lunch box addition or an ideal meal with a salad.

1. Preheat the oven to 190°C/Fan 170°C/Gas 5. Line a 12-hole muffin tin with cases (use silicone muffin cases, if possible).

2. Place the grated courgette (zucchini) in a clean tea towel and squeeze out as much liquid as possible.

3. Mix the ricotta with the eggs in a large bowl until smooth, then add the flour, baking powder and salt. Mix again until thoroughly combined.

4. Fold in the grated courgette (zucchini), feta cheese, most of the pumpkin seeds and all the basil.

5. Divide between the muffin cases, sprinkle with the remaining seeds and bake for 25 minutes.

PER SERVING / 145 CALS / PROTEIN 8.5G / SUGAR 0.9G / FIBRE 2.1G / CARBS 11.4G

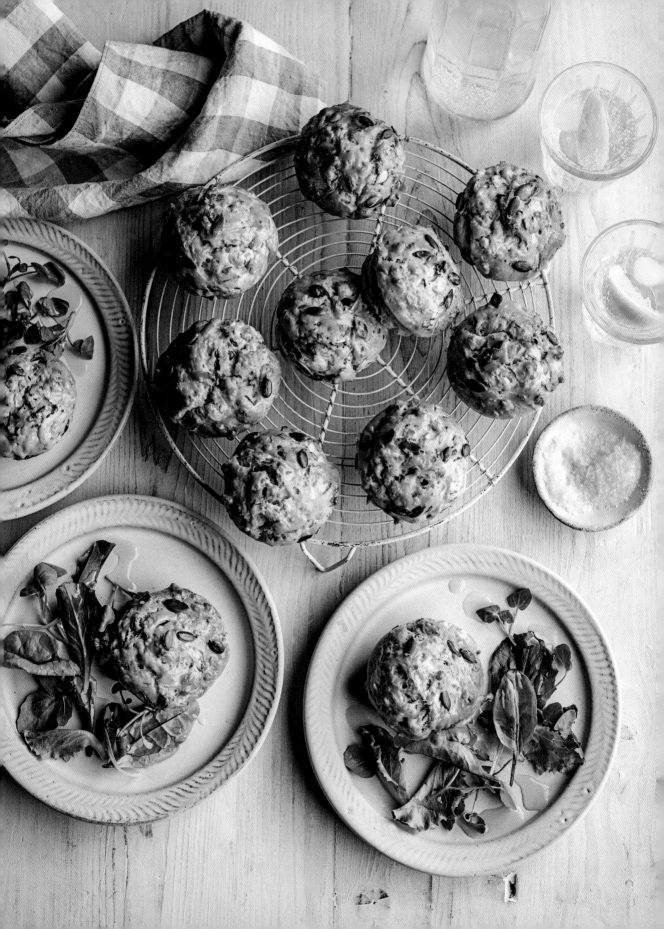

Chorizo and Parsley Muffins

MAKES	PREP	COOK
6	**15** mins	**15** mins

70g chorizo, finely chopped
55g full-fat cream cheese
4 medium free-range eggs
30g ground almonds
1 tsp baking powder
½ tsp salt
40g Cheddar, grated
10g parsley, leaves picked
  and roughly chopped
Zest of ½ lemon (optional)

Even a small portion of chorizo packs a punch of flavour, bringing a garlicky, paprika-flavoured kick, and making these high-protein muffins delicious and satisfying.

1. Preheat the oven to 190°C/Fan 170°C/Gas 5. Line a 12-hole muffin tin with 6 cases (use silicone muffin cases, if possible).

2. Place the chorizo in a dry frying pan over a medium heat and fry for 3–4 minutes, stirring occasionally, until the chorizo is crispy. Transfer to a plate lined with kitchen roll and set aside.

3. Place the cream cheese, eggs, ground almonds, baking powder and salt in a medium bowl and whisk until smooth.

4. Stir in the Cheddar, parsley, cooked chorizo and lemon zest, if using, and spoon the mixture into the muffin cases. Bake in the oven for 15 minutes.

5. Serve warm or leave to cool on a wire rack.

PER SERVING / 181 CALS / PROTEIN 11.4G / SUGAR 0.7G / FIBRE 0.1G / CARBS 1.2G

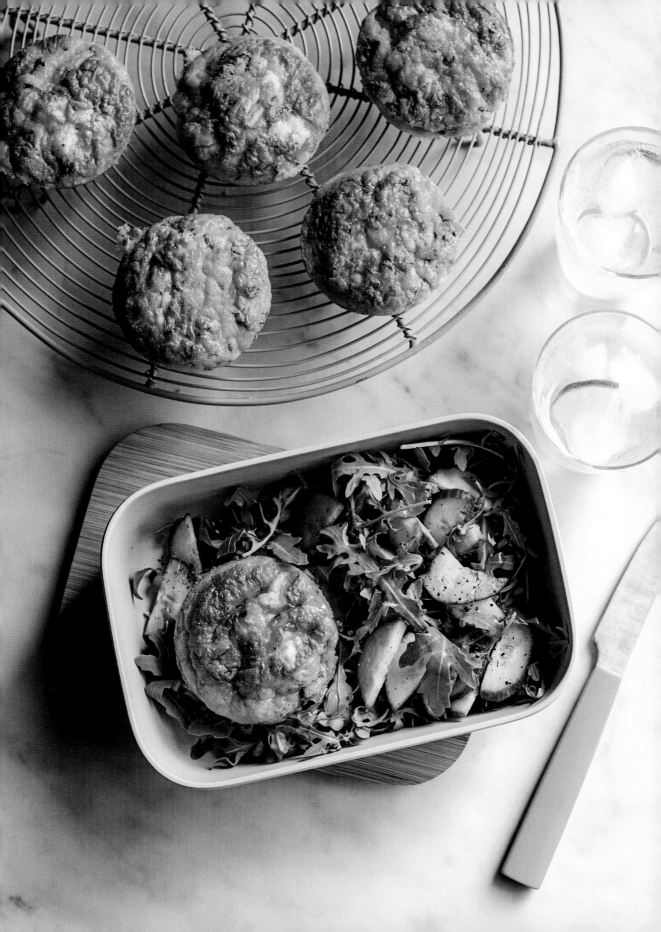

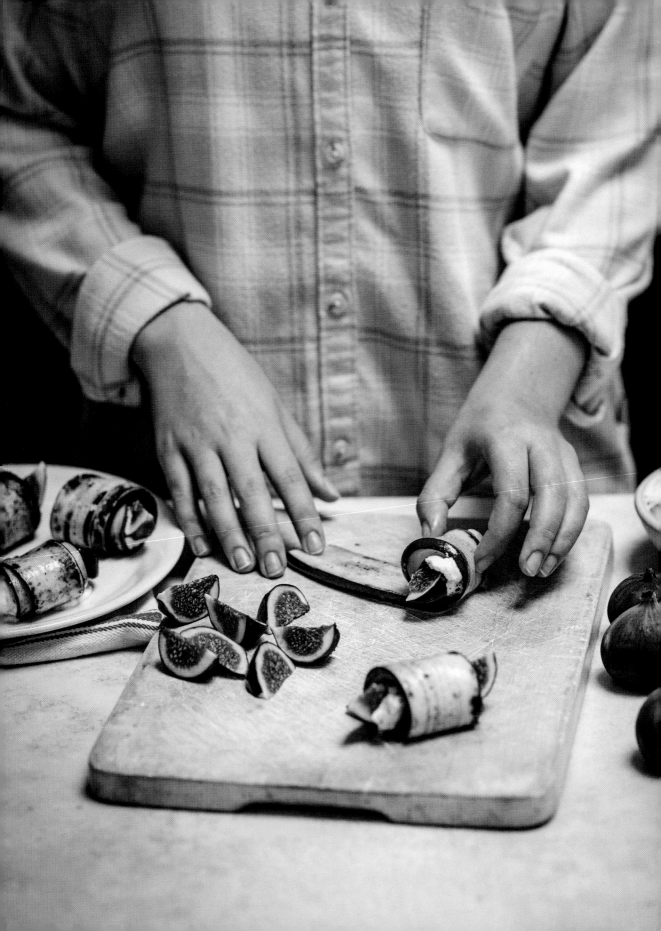

Savoury
Snacks

Fig and Goat's Cheese Rolls

MAKES
6

PREP
10
mins

COOK
2–3
mins

1 large courgette (zucchini)
   (about 250g)
1½ tsp olive oil
60g soft goat's cheese
10g blanched hazelnuts,
   finely chopped
2 small figs, each sliced into 6
   (70g prepared weight)

The nuts in this recipe create fantastic texture –
if you don't have hazelnuts, use walnuts, flaked
almonds, pistachios or pine nuts. Enjoy these rolls
straight away, or they will keep for a day in the
fridge to make a great grab-and-go snack.

1. Trim the courgette (zucchini) and slice into six
lengthways. The slices should be just under 0.5cm thick.
Season each slice with a pinch of salt and pepper.

2. Heat the oil in a large frying pan over a medium heat
and fry the courgette (zucchini) slices for 2 minutes on
each side, until golden. You may need to do this in batches.

3. Transfer the fried courgette (zucchini) to a plate lined
with kitchen roll to absorb the excess oil and leave to cool.

4. Meanwhile, mix the goat's cheese and hazelnuts together
in a small bowl with a pinch of salt and pepper.

5. To prepare the rolls, lay the fried courgette (zucchini)
slices on a flat surface. Place a teaspoon of nutty goat's
cheese at one end of the courgette (zucchini) slice, top
with two pieces of fig and roll tightly. Repeat with the
remaining ingredients.

PER SERVING / 65 CALS / PROTEIN 3.2G / SUGAR 1.9G / FIBRE 0.8G / CARBS 2G

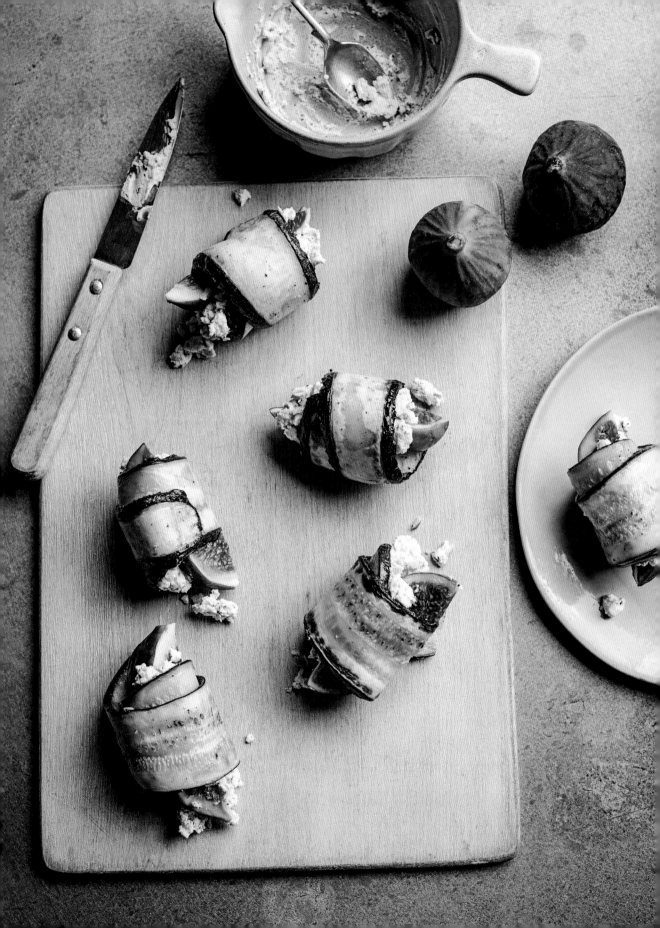

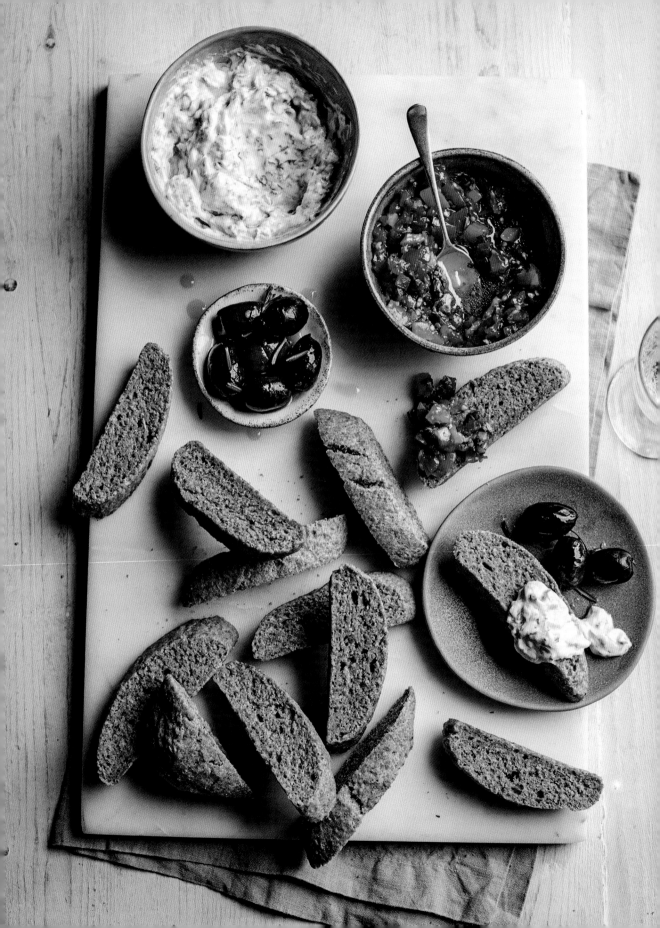

Parmesan Biscotti

MAKES **24** | **PREP** **20** mins | **COOK** **85** mins

250g wholegrain spelt flour
70g Parmesan, grated
1 tbsp ground black pepper
1 tsp baking powder
1 tsp salt
85g butter, softened
2 medium free-range eggs
125ml full-fat milk

COOK'S TIP
The biscotti should crisp up further as they cool. They keep well in an airtight container, or freeze in a sealed bag. If you want to crisp them up again, just pop them in a medium oven for 10 minutes.

Made with nutritious ancient grains, these cheesy savoury biscotti have a wonderful nutty, sweet and salty umami flavour. They are easy to make, but will need some attention while cooking as biscotti means 'twice baked'. Eat them on their own, serve with dips or scatter on soups and salads.

1. Preheat the oven to 180°C/Fan 160°C/Gas 4. Line a baking tray with non-stick baking paper.

2. Mix all the dry ingredients together in a medium bowl, then add the butter, eggs and milk. Stir together well until you have a sticky dough.

3. Scrape the dough out on to a generously floured work surface and shape into a rough ball using floured hands. Divide the dough in two, then shape each half into a log, approximately 25cm long and slightly flat on top. Transfer the dough to the prepared tray and bake for 25 minutes until just golden and firm.

4. Remove from the oven and leave to cool on a wire rack for 10 minutes. Reduce the oven temperature to 160°C/Fan 140°C/Gas 3.

5. Cut each log into 12 diagonal slices with a bread knife (they should be approximately 2cm wide). Place the slices back on the tray and return to the oven for 30 minutes on each side, until beginning to brown and crisp.

6. Leave to cool on a wire rack.

––––

PER SERVING / 86 CALS / PROTEIN 3.2G / SUGAR 0.4G / FIBRE 1 1G / CARBS 7.3G

Cheesy Biscuits with Rosemary

MAKES **20**

PREP **30** mins

COOK **10–15** mins

100g Parmesan, grated
100g Cheddar, grated
100g ground almonds
50g mixed seeds
1 sprig rosemary, leaves picked
  and finely chopped (1 level
  dessertspoon)
1 medium or large free-range
  egg white, lightly whisked

COOK'S TIP
The biscuits can be kept
in a container in the fridge
for up to a week or frozen.
They are best eaten warm,
though, so reheat for a few
minutes before serving if
they've been in the fridge
or freezer. You can use other
robust herbs, such as thyme
or sage, instead of rosemary.
This dough would also work
well cooked as a traybake,
then sliced into cheesy
snack bars. You would
need to increase the
cooking time, however.

Ideal for a savoury snack or as a lunch on the run.
Being high in protein, natural fat and fibre they
will also keep you full for longer. A treat that
shouldn't spike blood sugars!

1. Preheat the oven to 170°C/Fan 150°C/Gas 3½.
Line a large baking tray with non-stick baking paper.

2. Mix all the ingredients except the egg white in
a medium bowl.

3. Add the egg white and, using a wooden spoon, mix
vigorously to form a slightly crumbly dough. If it's too
crumbly, add ½ tablespoon of water and mix again
until it holds together.

4. With a dessertspoon in one hand, use your other hand
to scoop the mixture and press it firmly into the spoon
until it is almost level, then tip it out and place the
biscuit on the prepared tray.

5. Press the biscuit with a fork to achieve a thickness
of around 0.5–1cm. Repeat with the remaining dough
to make 20 biscuits. Bake for 10–12 minutes, checking
every few minutes, until they are light golden brown around
the edges. Transfer carefully to a wire rack
and leave to cool.

PER SERVING / 88 CALS / PROTEIN 5.1G / SUGAR 0.3G / FIBRE 0.2G / CARBS 0.6G

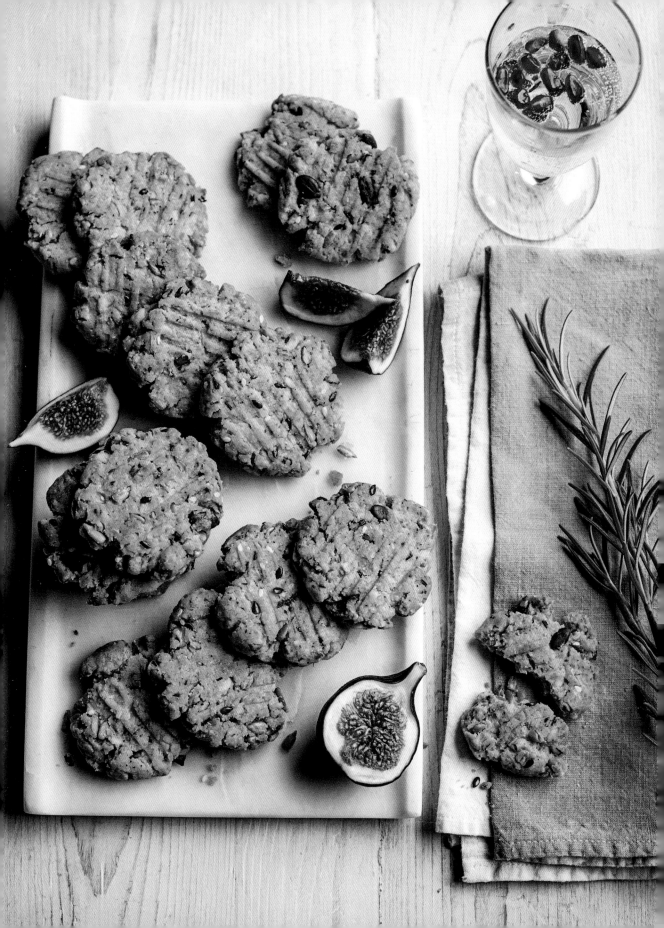

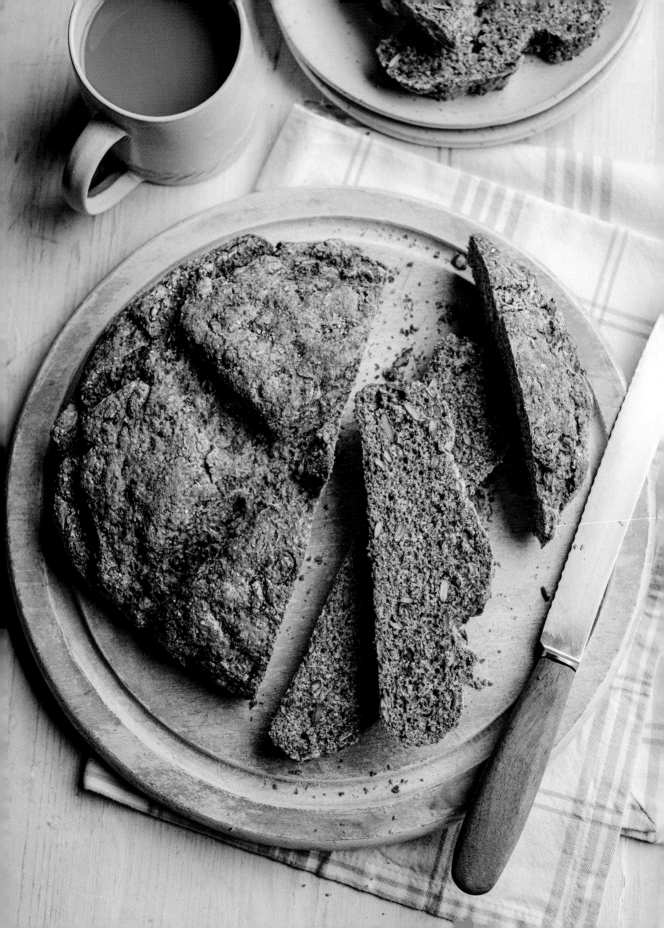

Seeded Spelt Soda Bread

MAKES	PREP	COOK
10	**10** mins	**30–35** mins

300g wholegrain spelt flour
1½ tsp bicarbonate of soda
1 tsp sea salt
80g pumpkin seeds
300ml full-fat natural yoghurt,
    or dairy-free equivalent
1 tbsp maple syrup

Soda bread is one of the easiest breads to make and, by using wholegrain spelt, it has plenty of fibre as well as protein. You could try using other ancient grains. As traditional buttermilk is hard to come by, we have used live natural yoghurt in this recipe, which behaves exactly the same. Best to eat in moderation if you are on a 800–1000 calorie fast day.

1. Preheat the oven to 200°C/Fan 180°C/Gas 6. Line a baking tray with non-stick baking paper.

2. Mix together the flour, bicarbonate of soda, sea salt and pumpkin seeds in a bowl. Make a well in the centre and pour in the yoghurt and maple syrup. Gently mix everything together to form a soft, sticky dough.

3. Turn the dough out on to a floured work surface and gently knead so that it forms a round loaf. Place the loaf on the prepared baking tray and shape it so that it is roughly 15cm wide and about 2.5cm deep. Cut a cross into the top, about 1cm deep, with a sharp knife and bake for 30–35 minutes, until it sounds hollow when tapped underneath.

4. Leave to cool on a wire rack. Cut into 10 slices to serve.

———

PER SERVING / 183 CALS / PROTEIN 7.7G / SUGAR 3.9G / FIBRE 3.6G / CARBS 24.6G

Classic Mug Bread

SERVES	PREP	COOK
2	**5** mins	**2** mins

1 level tbsp salted butter
   (or olive oil)
1 heaped tbsp flaxseed
3 heaped tbsp ground almonds
1 level tbsp seeds of your choice
   (such as pumpkin, sunflower
   or linseed)
1 tsp baking powder
1 small free-range egg

COOK'S TIP
Don't be disconcerted if you find a few holes in the bread when you turn it out of the mug. It is best eaten on the same day, although you can slice it and freeze any extra portions for toast.

This remarkable, instant, high-protein and high-fibre keto bread is cooked in the microwave in a mug in less than 5 minutes. It can be used as a breakfast muffin, as the base for an open sandwich or topped with scrambled egg for a delicious breakfast. It also makes satisfying toast. One of my favourites.

1. Place the butter in a mug and melt in the microwave for 8–10 seconds. Use a spatula to spread the butter all around the inside of the mug. Or coat in the olive oil, if using.

2. Add the rest of the ingredients to the mug with a pinch of salt and mix vigorously to make sure everything is well combined. Cook in the microwave for about 60–90 seconds.

3. Remove from the microwave and tap the top – if it's firm and springy, it's ready. If it's soft, return it to the microwave for another 10 seconds at a time, until firm.

4. Turn it upside down, tap to remove it from the mug, and place on a wire rack to cool. Cut into circular slices to serve.

PER SERVING / 320 CALS / PROTEIN 12.8G / SUGAR 1.1G / FIBRE 2.2G / CARBS 3.6G

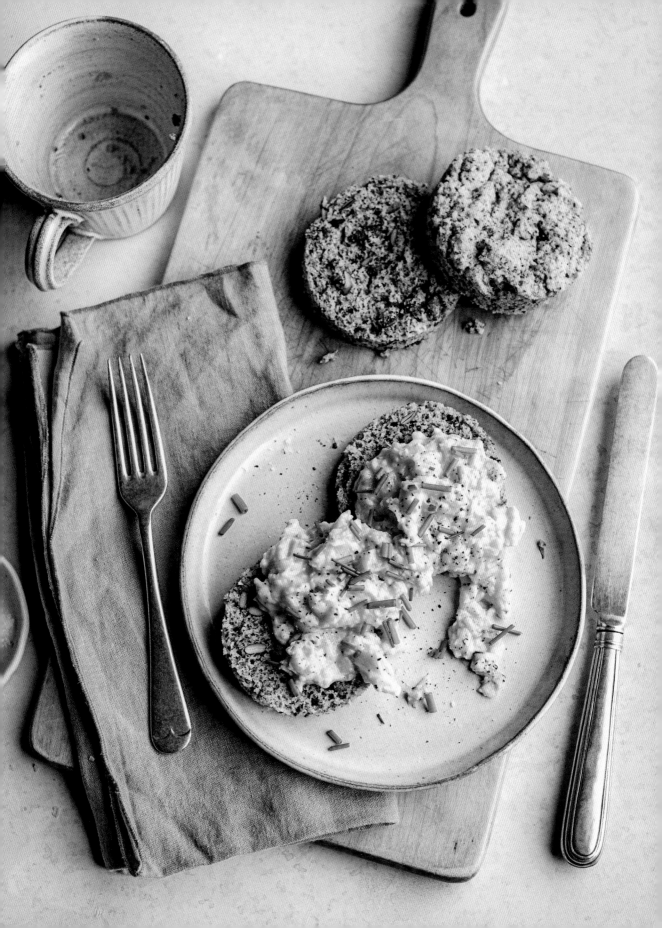

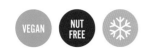

VEGAN   NUT FREE

Bird Seed Crackers

MAKES | **PREP** | **COOK**
12 | **20** mins | **30** mins

3 tbsp wholegrain spelt flour (or wholegrain buckwheat flour)
275g mixed seeds
2 tbsp chia seeds
1–2 tsp flaked sea salt

These crunchy, high-fibre crackers have a satisfying savoury toasted flavour and make a great alternative to serve with dips or to crumble into soups or scatter on salads.

1. Preheat the oven to 180°C/Fan 160°C/Gas 4 and line a 33×23cm baking tray with non-stick baking paper.

2. Mix all the ingredients in a medium bowl along with plenty of ground black pepper.

3. Pour in 200ml of water and mix well. Leave to settle for about 15 minutes; it will thicken and feel tacky.

4. Tip the mixture on to the prepared baking tray and use a spatula to spread it out in a thin, even layer. Score it lightly with criss-cross lines, ready to separate into about 12 crackers. Bake for about 15-20 minutes, until starting to turn golden in places, then turn the crackers over and cook for about 15 minutes more. Don't overcook the crackers or they will taste bitter. Turn off the oven and leave to dry out in the oven for an hour or two.

5. Once cool, store in sealed container for up to 1 week. If they get soft, you can pop them in the oven for 5 minutes to crisp up.

———

PER SERVING / 154 CALS / PROTEIN 5.5G / SUGAR 0.3G / FIBRE 3G / CARBS 6G

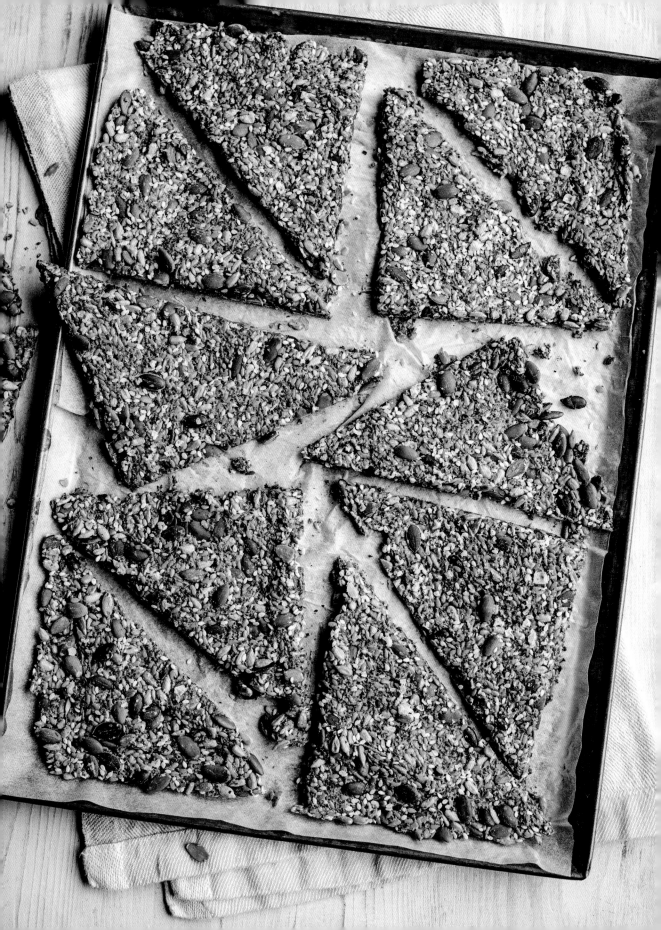

Fruit 'Blinis'

MAKES **4** | **PREP** **8–10** mins

These fruit-based 'blinis' make a lovely change from the stodgy, rubbery discs we usually call blinis. They make fabulous starters or nibbles to be shared and are unlikely to spike blood sugars too.

Pear with Blue Cheese, Hazelnut and Peppadew Peppers

1 small pear, core removed
   and sliced into 4 discs
   (each about 0.5cm thick)
½ tsp lemon juice
2 slices blue cheese, each slice
   halved (30g total weight),
   or dairy-free equivalent
10g hazelnuts,
   roughly chopped
12 Peppadew (or piquanté)
   peppers

1. Brush each side of pear with a little lemon juice to stop it from browning.

2. Top each slice with some blue cheese, then press the chopped hazelnuts into the cheese so they don't fall off.

3. Place 3 Peppadew peppers on top of each slice and season with salt and pepper.

_____

PER SERVING / 135 CALS / PROTEIN 4.6G / SUGAR 8.6G / FIBRE 2.5G / CARBS 8.7G

Apple with Cheddar and Relish

1 small apple, cored and
   sliced into 4 discs
   (each about 0.5cm thick)
½ tsp lemon juice
15g walnuts, finely chopped
3 sprigs of parsley, leaves
   picked and finely chopped
1 tsp apple cider vinegar
2 slices Cheddar, each slice
   halved (30g total weight),
   or dairy-free equivalent

1. Brush each side of apple with a little lemon juice
to stop it from browning.

2. In a small bowl, mix the walnuts, parsley and apple
cider vinegar. Season with a pinch of salt and pepper.

3. Lay a slice of Cheddar on top of each apple slice
and top with the walnut relish.

———

PER SERVING / 191 CALS / PROTEIN 5.7G / SUGAR 16G / FIBRE 3.2G / CARBS 16.1G

Pear with Smoked Mackerel Pâté

1 small pear, core removed
   and sliced into 4 discs
   (each about 0.5cm thick)
1 tsp lemon juice
1 small smoked mackerel
   fillet, skin removed
   (50g prepared weight)
1 tbsp full-fat cream cheese
2 sprigs of dill, leaves picked
   and roughly chopped

1. Using half the lemon juice, brush each side of pear
to stop it from browning.

2. Place the mackerel and remaining lemon juice
in a small bowl and mash to break into small pieces.
Add the cream cheese, dill and a pinch of salt and
pepper, and mix until combined.

3. Divide the mackerel pâté between the slices of
pear to serve.

———

PER SERVING / 136 CALS / PROTEIN 6.1G / SUGAR 8.5G / FIBRE 2G / CARBS 8.5G

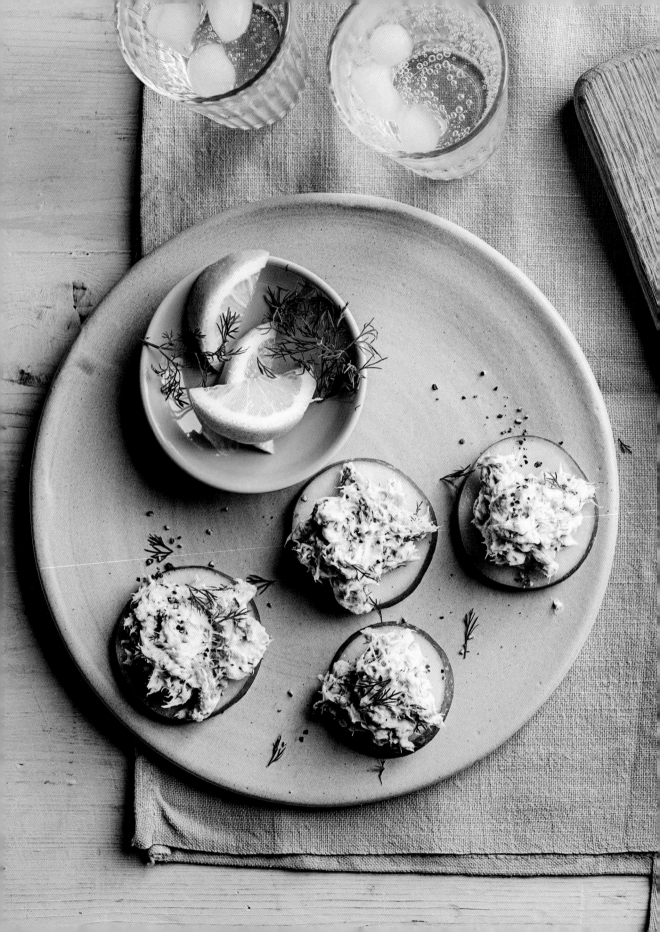

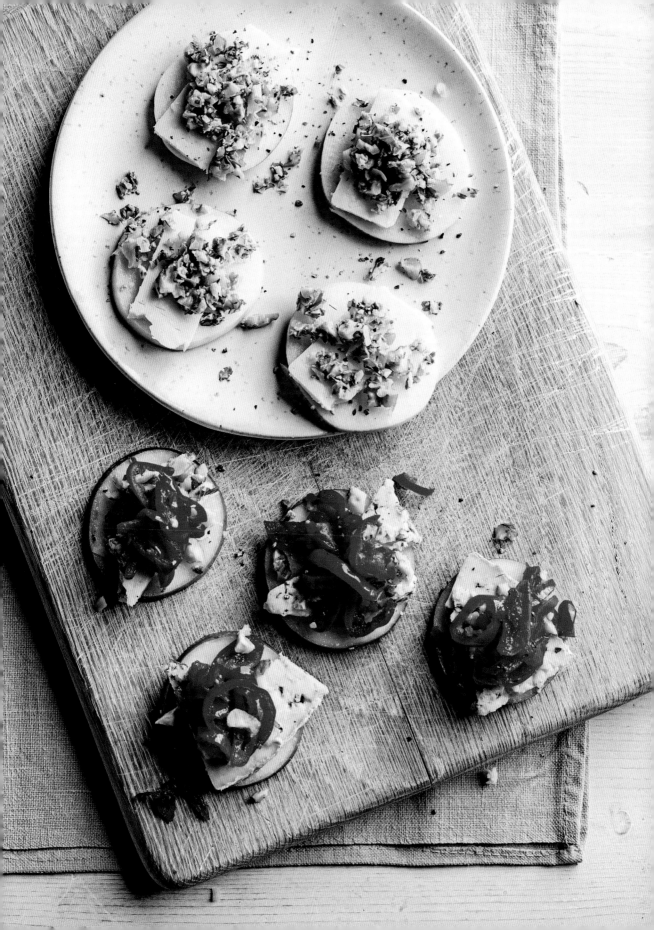

Beetroot Blinis with Cream Cheese, Smoked Salmon and Dill

MAKES	PREP	COOK
4	**10** mins	**6** mins

30g wholegrain
buckwheat flour
½ tsp baking powder
50g full-fat Greek yoghurt
1 medium free-range egg
20g Parmesan, finely grated
1 cooked beetroot,
finely diced (50g)
1 tsp olive oil
4 tbsp full-fat cream cheese
200g smoked salmon,
divided into 4
4 sprigs of dill,
roughly chopped
black pepper, to serve
lemon slices, to serve

Enjoy this omega-3-rich salmon blini, that is not only delicious and colourful but also brings the added benefits of beetroot, enhancing circulation and boosting exercise performance.

1. Place the flour, baking powder, yoghurt, egg and Parmesan in a bowl with a pinch of salt and pepper and mix until smooth. Fold in the beetroot and set aside.

2. Heat the oil in a large frying pan over a medium heat and, when hot, use all the batter to spoon four blinis into the pan (or do two at a time if your frying pan is too small to fit four). Fry for 1½ minutes, flip over and cook for 1½ minutes on the other side.

3. Transfer to a plate lined with kitchen roll and allow to cool slightly.

4. When ready to serve, top each blini with a tablespoon of cream cheese, a slice of smoked salmon and a sprinkling of dill and black pepper and serve with lemon slices.

PER SERVING / 232 CALS / PROTEIN 17.2G / SUGAR 2.3G / FIBRE 0.6G / CARBS 8.6G

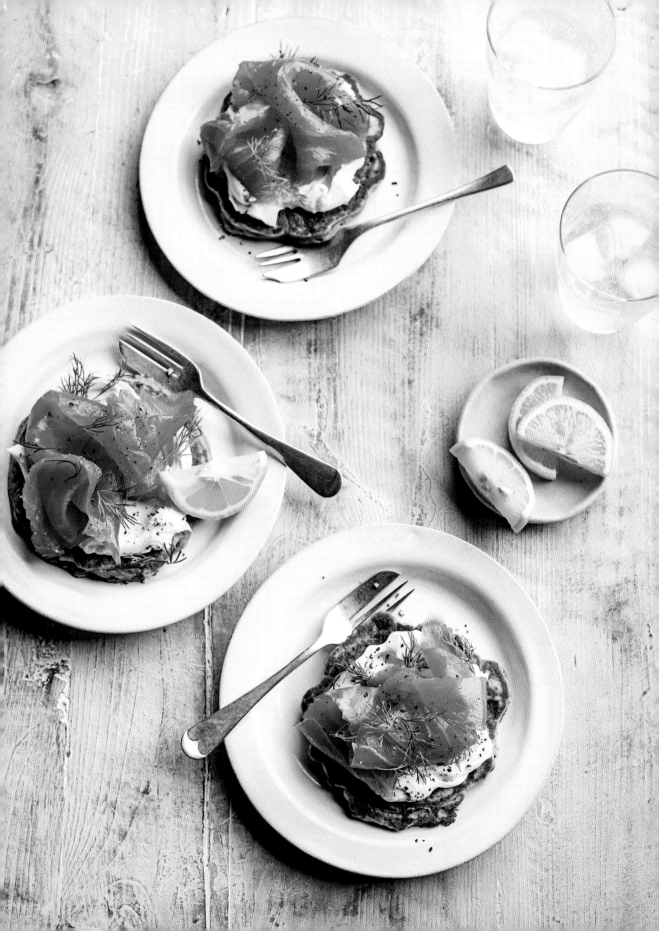

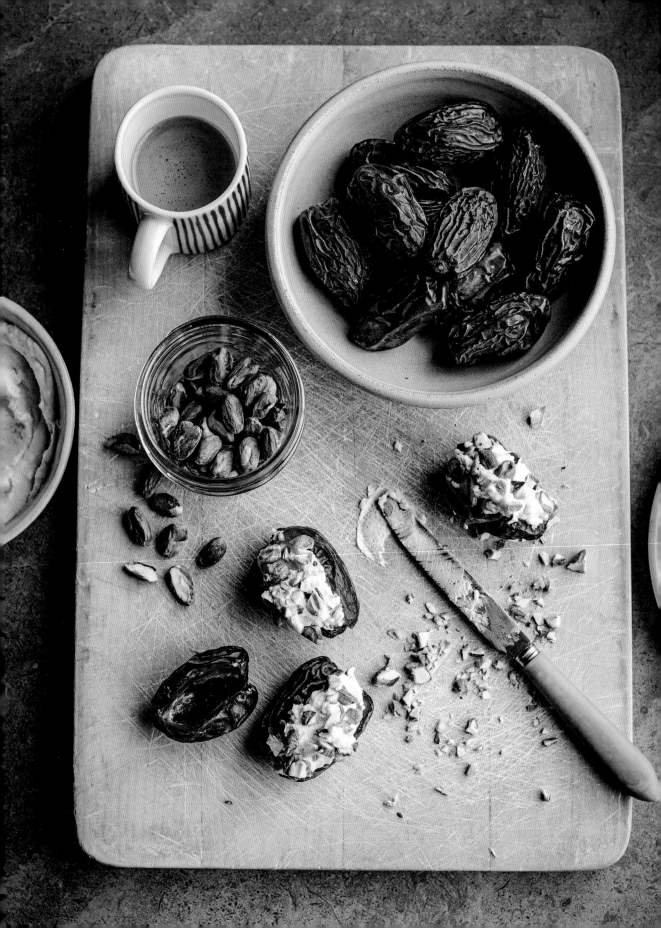

Ricotta and Pistachio Stuffed Dates

MAKES
1

PREP
2
mins

1 medjool date
1 rounded tsp ricotta
 (or full-fat cream cheese),
 or dairy-free equivalent
A few shelled pistachios,
 chopped

An instant and delicious treat. The sweetness of the date contrasts with the cream and crunch of the filling. Rich in fibre to reduce any sugar spike, dates are 'nature's toffee'. Combining the dates with healthy fats flattens the sugar curve too.

1. Split the date open and remove the stone.

2. Fill the cavity with the ricotta or cream cheese, then sprinkle with the chopped pistachios. Press the nuts gently into the cheese to secure.

――――

PER SERVING / 87 CALS / PROTEIN 1.9G / SUGAR 11.8G / FIBRE 1.5G / CARBS 12.7G

Mediterranean Cheesy Squashed Scones

MAKES | **PREP** | **COOK**
14 | **10** mins | **25** mins

200g feta cheese, crumbled
1 ball of mozzarella,
    broken into small pieces
120g wholegrain spelt flour
1 tsp baking powder
1 heaped tsp dried oregano
1 tsp garlic granules
2 medium free-range eggs
60ml olive oil
60ml full-fat milk

COOK'S TIP
These scones are
naturally salty, due
to the feta, so there's
no need to add salt
to the dough.

The tangy cheese and herbs make these scones an ideal companion to soup, or a tomato or leafy green salad. They also work well in a lunch box. Gut-friendly feta adds protein and calcium. These are best served warm.

1. Preheat the oven to 200°C/Fan 180°C/Gas 6.
Line a large baking tray with non-stick baking paper.

2. Place all the ingredients in a bowl and mix well.

3. Divide the mixture into 14 spoonfuls and transfer to the prepared tray. Bake for 25 minutes or until golden.

4. Serve warm or leave to cool on a wire rack and store in an airtight tin or freeze. Warm in the oven as needed.

———

PER SERVING / 132 CALS / PROTEIN 6.1G / SUGAR 0.5G / FIBRE 0.9G / CARBS 6.2G

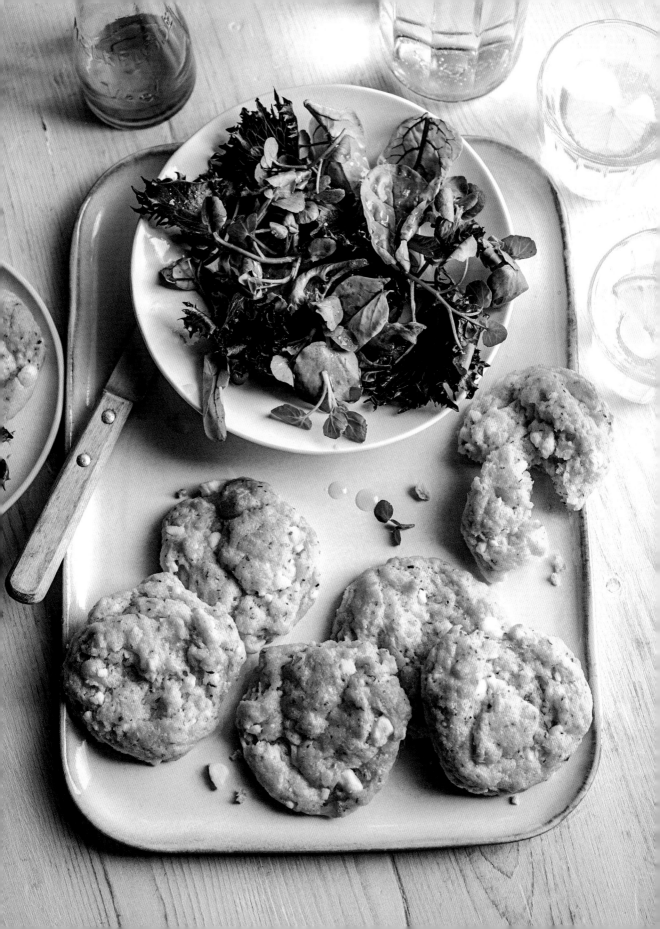

Savoury Parmesan Popcorn

SERVES | **PREP** | **COOK**
4 | **2** mins | **2** mins

1 tbsp plus 1 tsp olive oil
3 tbsp popcorn kernels
¼ tsp cayenne pepper
½ tsp garlic powder
10g Parmesan, or dairy-free
   equivalent, finely grated

Who said popcorn can't be a healthy treat? This mouthwatering, spiced, garlic- and Parmesan-flavoured popcorn is irresistible, and the natural fat and fibre help to keep sugars down.

1. Place 1 tablespoon of the olive oil in a large saucepan with the popcorn kernels and cover with a tightly fitting lid. Place the saucepan over a high heat and pop the corn for 1½–2 minutes. When the popping begins to slow, turn off the heat and leave the pan for a few seconds longer until the popping stops.

2. Transfer the popcorn to a large bowl and set aside to cool a little.

3. Drizzle the remaining olive oil over the popcorn and toss well. Sprinkle with the cayenne pepper, garlic powder, grated Parmesan and a generous pinch of salt and toss again to coat. Serve straight away or store in an airtight container for up to 2 days.

PER SERVING / 74 CALS / PROTEIN 0.9G / SUGAR 0.1G / FIBRE 0.2G / CARBS 7.8G

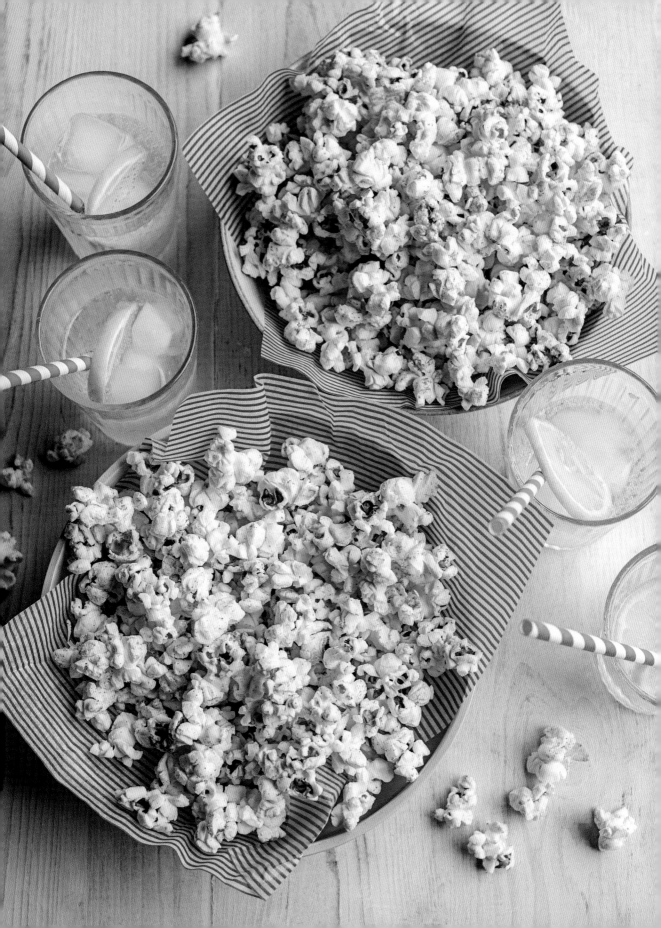

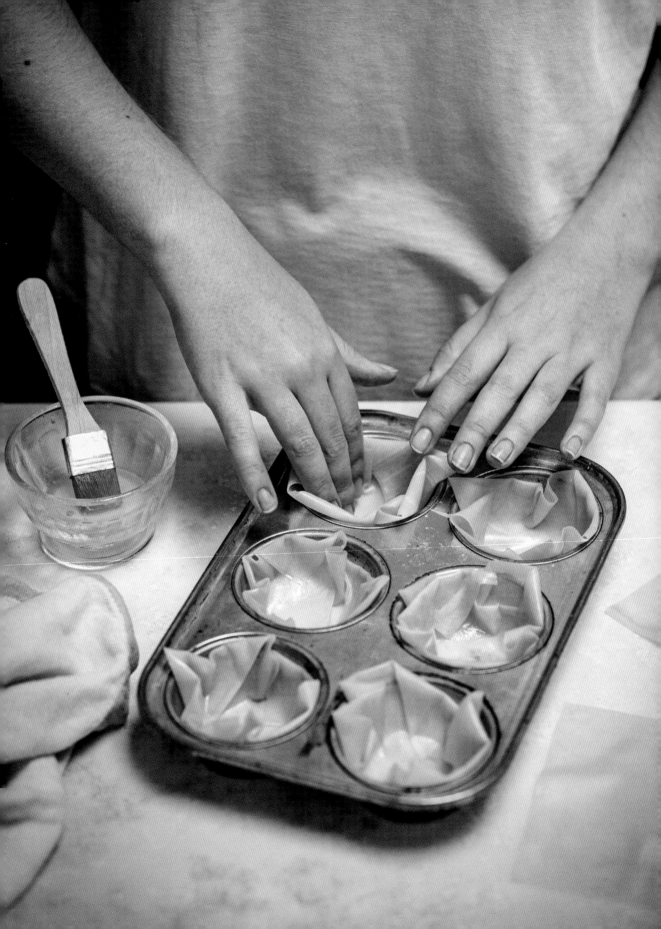

Oven Bakes

Cheat Custard Tarts

SERVES | **PREP** | **COOK**
4 | **15** mins | **8–10** mins

1 sheet filo pastry, cut into
   8 equal squares
25g butter, melted
125g mascarpone cheese
35ml full-fat milk
1 tsp vanilla paste
   (or 2 tsp vanilla extract)
Zest of ½ lemon
½ tsp honey

COOK'S TIP
The pastry cases will keep
in an airtight container
for about a week.

Missing pastry tarts? Well, these are healthy, light custard tarts for all the family. Use silicone muffin cases, if you can. As they are non-stick, you'll get an even bake and the cases come in glorious colours. Double the quantities for a crowd.

1. Preheat the oven to 200°C/Fan 180°C/Gas 6.

2. Brush one square of filo with melted butter, then brush another and lay them on top of each other. Press them into a silicone muffin case, folding the overhanging pieces back into the muffin case, so that the pastry is fully lining the case – don't worry if the pastry overlaps and is thicker in some places. Continue with the remaining pastry and butter until you have four lined muffin cases.

3. Place the muffin cases on a baking tray and bake in the oven for 8–10 minutes, or until the pastry is golden and crisp. Set aside to cool slightly.

4. Remove the pastry cases from their muffin cases and place them on a piece of kitchen roll to absorb the excess melted butter.

5. Meanwhile, mix the mascarpone, milk, vanilla, lemon zest and honey in a small bowl until smooth. Divide the mixture between the cooled pastry cases and level the tops.

6. Serve the tarts as they are or with fresh berries.

PER SERVING / 223 CALS / PROTEIN 2.6G / SUGAR 3.4G / FIBRE 0.3G / CARBS 8.8G

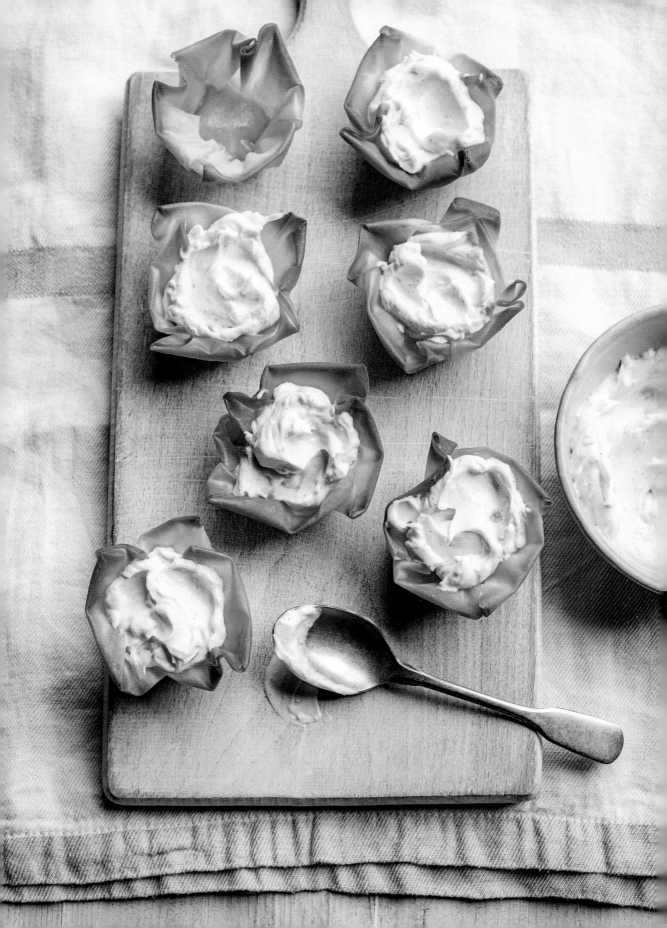

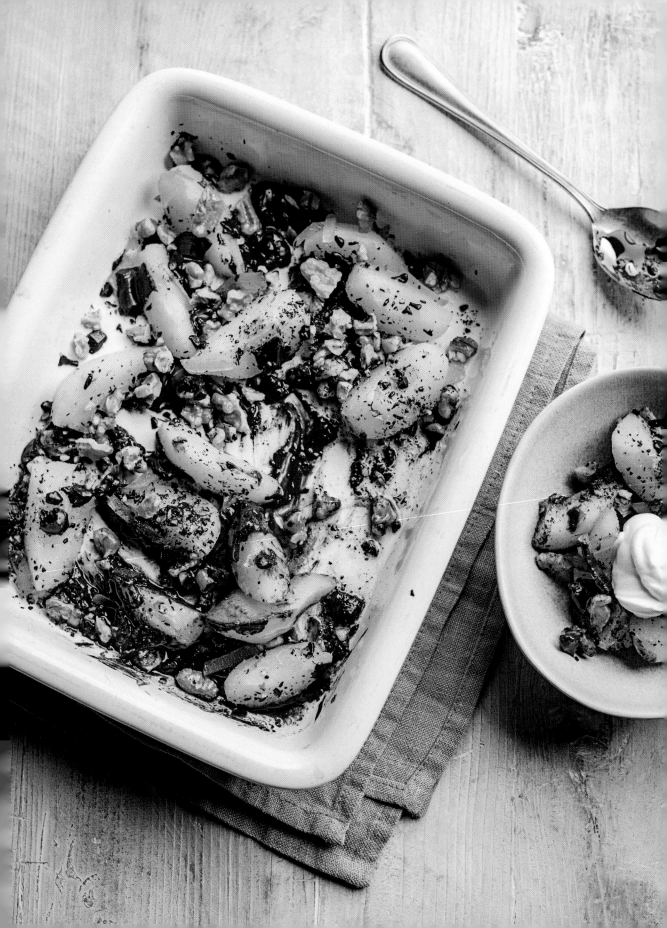

Quick Baked Pears with Ginger and Walnuts

SERVES | **PREP** | **COOK**
4 | **10** mins | **15** mins

1 tbsp coconut oil, melted
1 × 400g tin pears in fruit juice
1 ball of stem ginger in syrup,
    drained and finely chopped
50g dark chocolate (at least
    70%), roughly chopped
30g walnuts, roughly broken

We often eat tinned fruit – no peeling required, ready sliced and easy to assemble. I recommend you keep tinned fruit in the cupboard, too, as it is generally just as nutritious as fresh fruit and will always be on hand to make an easy dessert. Go for the fruit in fruit juice, rather than in syrup.

1. Preheat the oven to 190°C/Fan 170°C/Gas 5. Use some of the coconut oil to grease a small baking dish.

2. Drain the pears and slice each half into 3 wedges. Layer the wedges in the baking dish, slightly overlapping.

3. Drizzle the remaining coconut oil and scatter the chopped ginger over the top of the pears. Bake in the oven for 10 minutes.

4. Remove from the oven and scatter the chocolate chunks and walnuts over the pears. Return them to the oven for a further 5 minutes, until golden brown in places.

5. Serve as they are or with a tablespoon of full-fat Greek yoghurt, if you like.

PER SERVING / 354 CALS / PROTEIN 4.2G / SUGAR 31.3G / FIBRE 4G / CARBS 31.3G

Fig 'n' Nut Granola

SERVES	PREP	COOK
12	**15** mins	**25** mins

4 tbsp coconut oil (or butter)
2 tbsp honey
2 tsp ground cinnamon
8 large soft figs, stalks removed and diced (about 120g prepared weight)
1 medium free-range egg white, whisked with a fork
200g rolled oats
200g mixed nuts

This nutty, seedy granola is delicately flavoured, wonderfully crunchy and a little goes a long way. Enjoy it with full-fat Greek yoghurt for breakfast or scatter it on top of fruity puddings. Add an extra tablespoon of honey when making the paste if you have a sweet tooth. Don't overcook the granola, or it may taste bitter.

1. Preheat the oven to 170°C/Fan 150°C/Gas 3½. Line a large tray with non-stick baking paper.

2. Place the coconut oil or butter in a small pan over a gentle heat. Once melted, remove from the heat and stir in the honey, cinnamon and figs. Use the back of a spoon to mix to a paste, then leave to cool.

3. When the mixture is close to room temperature, stir in the egg white.

4. Meanwhile, combine the oats and nuts in a medium bowl with a generous pinch of salt. Pour the figgy paste on to the oats and nuts and mix well.

5. Scatter the granola evenly over the prepared tray and place in the oven for about 20 minutes, stirring halfway, until only slightly golden brown in places.

6. Leave to cool and crisp up on the tray before storing in an airtight jar for up to a few weeks.

_____

PER SERVING / 216 CALS / PROTEIN 6.6G / SUGAR 7.4G / FIBRE 2.2G / CARBS 18.6G

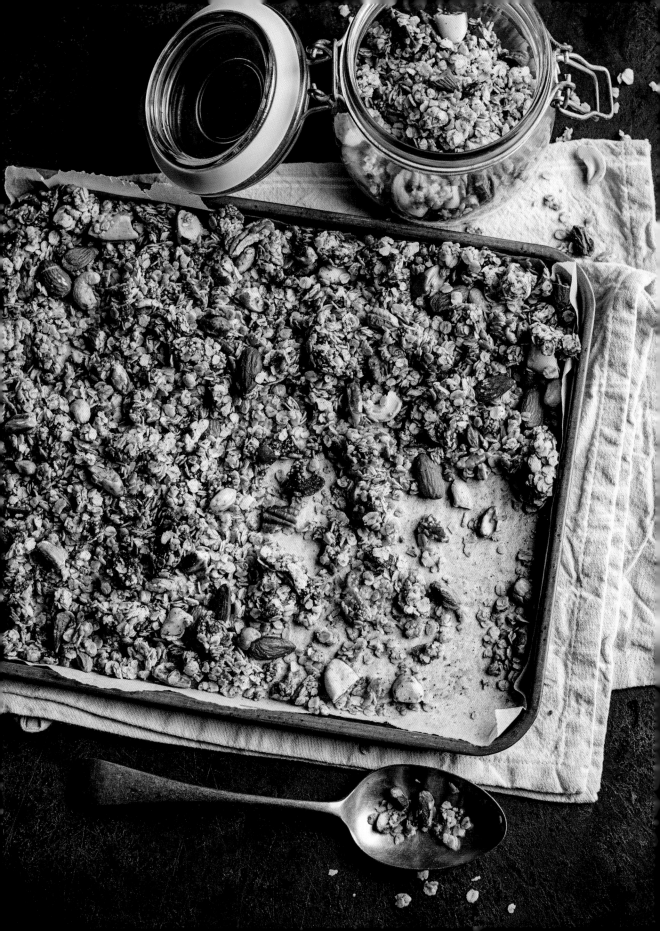

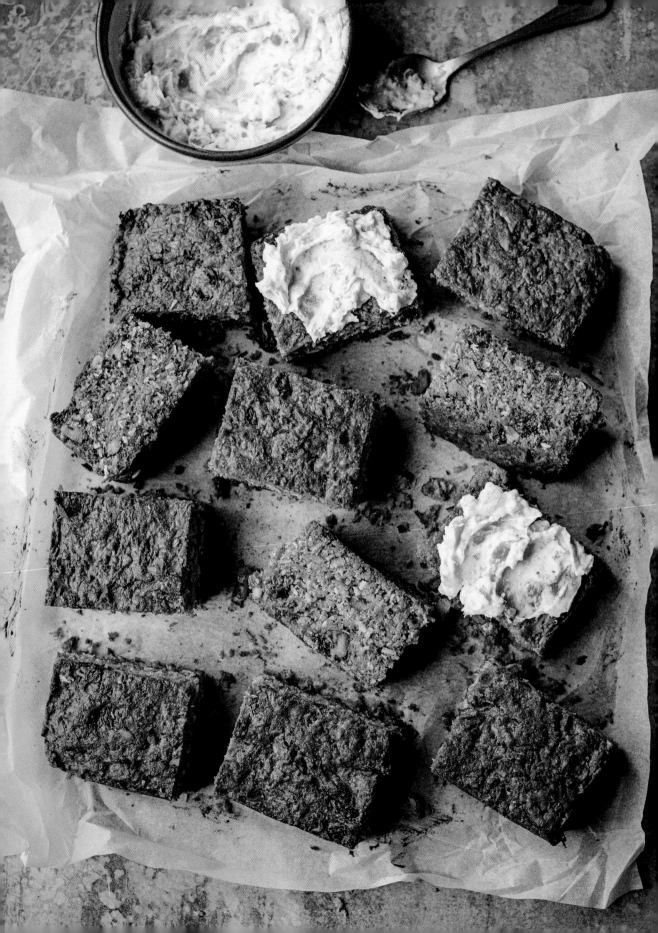

Cardamom Carrot Cake

SERVES	PREP	COOK
12	**25** mins	**60–75** mins

320g carrots, grated

80g soft pitted dates, finely
  chopped (or 1 tbsp honey)

3 large free-range eggs

150g coconut oil, melted

Zest of 1 orange

1 tsp ground cardamom
  (or seeds from 8
  cardamom pods)

160g wholegrain buckwheat
  flour (or gluten-free flour)

1 tbsp baking powder

½ tsp fine sea salt

120g desiccated coconut

120g walnuts, chopped

100g sultanas

COOK'S TIP

The cake will keep for
3 days, or cut it into slices
when it is cold and freeze.

A deliciously moist vegetable- and nut-based cake.
The wholegrain buckwheat flour brings extra fibre
to boost your microbiome. The cardamom gives this
cake a wonderful, warming aroma. Try this with the
Apricot Cream Cheese Frosting on page 112.

1. Preheat the oven to 170°C/Fan 150°C/Gas 3½.
Line a 20cm cake tin with non-stick baking paper.

2. Add the carrots, dates, eggs, coconut oil and orange
zest to a large bowl and mix well. Stir in the cardamom,
flour, baking powder, salt and desiccated coconut,
reserving 1 tablespoon of coconut for decoration,
and blitz the mixture briefly with a hand-held blender.
Vigorously stir in the walnuts and sultanas.

3. Pour the mixture into the prepared tin and bake
for 60–75 minutes, until a skewer inserted into the
centre comes out clean. If the top is browning before
the centre is done, cover the cake with a piece of foil.
Scatter the reserved desiccated coconut over the
cake 5 minutes before removing it from the oven.

4. Remove from the oven and leave to cool in the tin
before turning out on to a wire rack.

5. Allow to cool fully before storing in an airtight container.

PER SERVING / 364 CALS / PROTEIN 6.2G / SUGAR 9.8G / FIBRE 3.9G / CARBS 21.1G

Orange and Pistachio Upside-down Cake

SERVES	PREP	COOK
8	15 mins	20–25 mins

½ tsp coconut oil, melted
1 large orange, peeled
   and cut into 5 slices
25g shelled pistachios,
   roughly chopped
6 dried apricots,
   roughly chopped
3 medium free-range eggs
100g full-fat Greek yoghurt,
   or dairy-free equivalent
70ml olive oil
1 tsp almond extract
2 tsp vanilla extract
200g ground almonds
2 tsp baking powder

COOK'S TIP
The cake freezes
well. When cooled,
just cut it into slices
before freezing.

There is something magical about an upside-down cake. There's also a hint of jeopardy! With the base of ground almonds, eggs and nuts, this indulgent high-protein cake will leave you satisfyingly full without spiking sugars.

1. Preheat the oven to 200°C/Fan 180°C/Gas 6. Line a 20cm square baking dish with non-stick baking paper. Brush the non-stick baking paper all over with the melted coconut oil, then lay the orange slices on the base of the tin. Scatter the pistachios around the orange slices and set aside.

2. Place the dried apricots, eggs, yoghurt, olive oil and almond and vanilla extracts in a food processor or blender and blitz until the apricots are broken up and the mixture is smooth.

3. Add the ground almonds, baking powder and a pinch of salt and mix until combined. Pour into the prepared tin, smooth the surface and bake in the oven for 20–25 minutes, or until golden and a skewer inserted into the centre comes out clean. Allow to cool slightly and tip out on to wire rack. Carefully remove the non-stick baking paper.

4. Slice and serve with Greek yoghurt or crème fraîche.

PER SERVING / 301 CALS / PROTEIN 11.1G / SUGAR 5.6G / FIBRE 0.8G / CARBS 6.6G

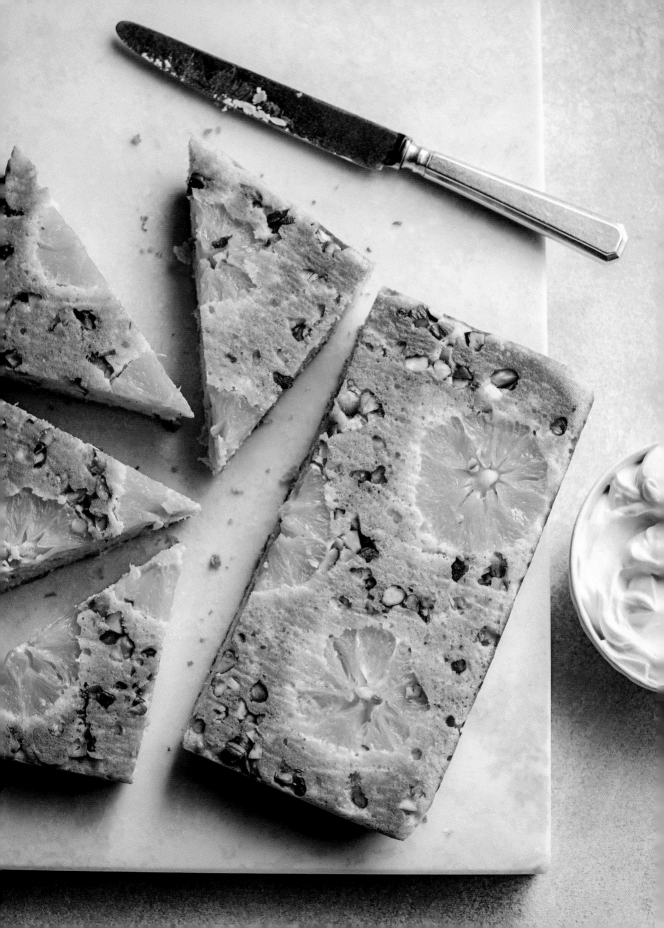

Earl Grey Tea Loaf with Apricot Cream Cheese Frosting

SERVES | **PREP** | **COOK**
10 | **15** mins | **40** mins

3 Earl Grey tea bags
250g ground almonds
2 tsp baking powder
75g sultanas
2 medium free-range eggs
75g coconut oil, melted
150g full-fat Greek yoghurt
2 tsp vanilla extract

For the Apricot Cream
Cheese Frosting
100g full-fat cream cheese
4 dried apricots, finely diced
3 tbsp full-fat Greek yoghurt
1 tbsp honey (optional)

COOK'S TIP
You could scatter one
diced apricot on top for
decoration, if you like.
The tea loaf freezes well.
Just wrap the slices
individually in non-stick
baking paper (without
frosting) and defrost
a slice at a time.

A fragrant black tea, scented with bergamot oils,
Earl Grey tea has been used for years thanks to its
health benefits. But it is not just here to sip elegantly,
it also works well to flavour cakes. Use ground tea
rather than leaves, which will otherwise need
grinding with a pestle and mortar.

1. Preheat the oven to 190°C/Fan 170°C/Gas 5.
Line a 900g loaf tin with non-stick baking paper.

2. Remove the tea from the tea bags and add to a medium
bowl with 2 tablespoons of water. Stir until combined.

3. Add the ground almonds, baking powder, sultanas,
eggs, coconut oil, yoghurt and vanilla extract to the bowl
and mix until combined and the tea is evenly distributed.

4. Transfer to the prepared loaf tin and bake for 40 minutes.
Check after 30 minutes to see if the surface is burning.
If it is, cover with foil. When ready, remove from the
oven and leave to cool in the tin.

5. To make the frosting, add the ingredients to a small
bowl and blitz using a hand-held blender. Spread the
frosting on top of the cooled cake.

6. Cut into 10 slices and store in an airtight container.

PER SERVING / 265 CALS / PROTEIN 8.3G / SUGAR 6.9G / FIBRE 0.5G / CARBS 7.7G

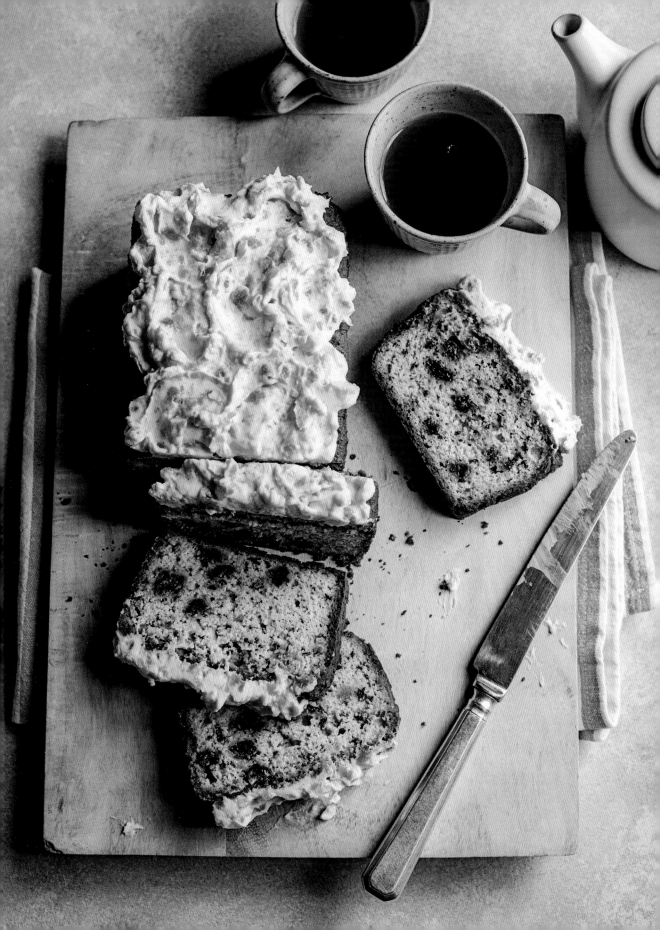

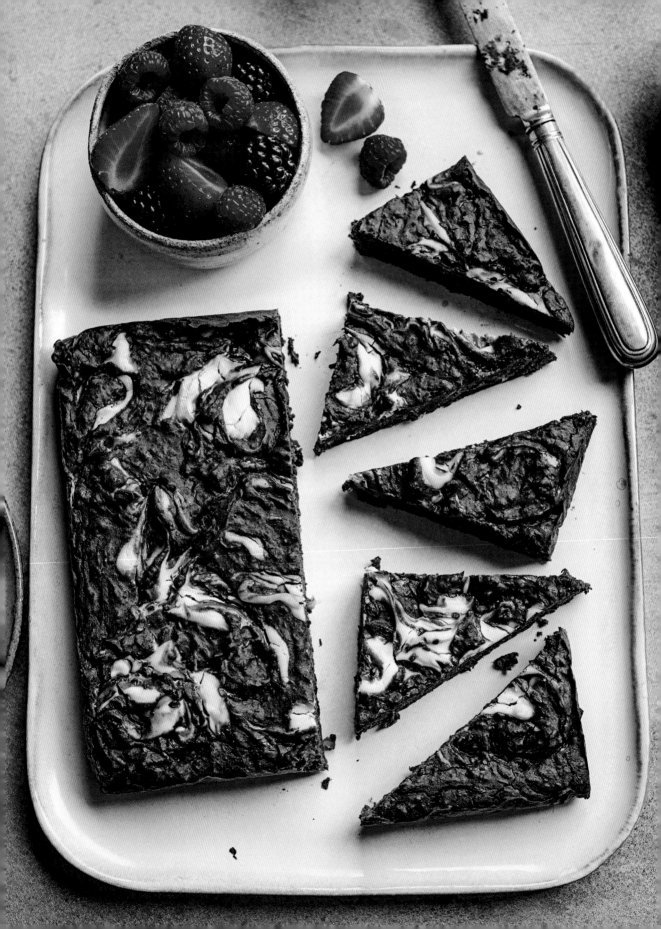

Chocolate Cheesecake Black Bean Brownies

MAKES
12

PREP
10 mins

COOK
20 mins

1 × 400g tin black beans, drained and rinsed
3 medium free-range eggs
100g soft pitted dates
3 tbsp unsweetened cocoa powder
3 tbsp coconut oil
2 tsp vanilla extract
30g dark chocolate chips
2 tbsp full-fat cream cheese, or dairy-free equivalent
1 tbsp honey

These brownies are a family favourite in Kathryn's house – dense and gooey in the centre and topped with a delicious cheesecake swirl. See if anyone can guess the main ingredient...

1. Preheat the oven to 190°C/Fan 170°C/Gas 5. Line a 20cm square cake tin with non-stick baking paper.

2. Place the black beans, eggs, dates, cocoa powder, coconut oil, 1 teaspoon of the vanilla extract and a pinch of salt in a food processor or blender and blitz for about 2 minutes, until really smooth.

3. Stir in the chocolate chips and pour the mixture into the prepared tin.

4. Mix the cream cheese, remaining vanilla extract and honey together in a small bowl until smooth. Swirl into the surface of the brownie mixture creating a marbled effect. Bake in the oven for 20 minutes.

5. Leave to cool in the tin, then slice into 12 to serve.

PER SERVING / 115 CALS / PROTEIN 4.3G / SUGAR 5.3G / FIBRE 2.8G / CARBS 7.2G

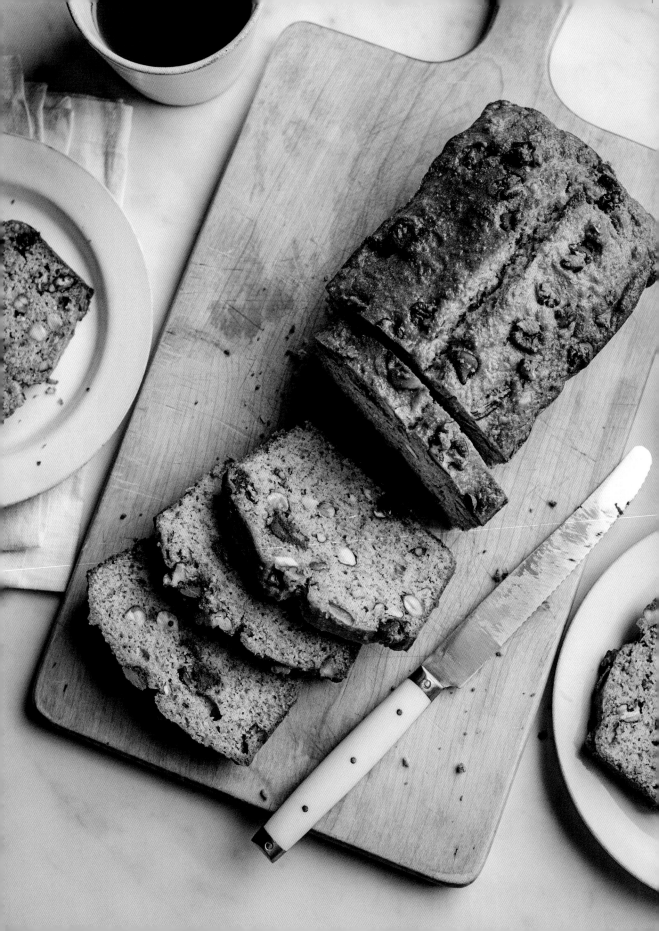

Chocolate Chip Banana Bread

SERVES	PREP	COOK
12	**15** mins	**50** mins

2–3 very ripe medium bananas
  (about 250g prepared weight),
  peeled and mashed
2 large free-range eggs, beaten
200g ground almonds
75g butter, melted
50g wholemeal
  self-raising flour
1 tsp ground mixed spice
1 tsp baking powder
75g mixed nuts,
  roughly chopped
60g dark chocolate chips

COOK'S TIP
The banana bread will
keep for 3 days, and it
freezes well. Just wrap
the slices individually in
non-stick baking paper
and defrost a slice at a time.

A popular baked treat, combining ripe bananas with chocolate chips in a moist loaf. Golden brown and crusted, with the bitter sweetness of the chocolate, this is the ultimate comfort food. But one that won't significantly spike your sugars, thanks to the ground almonds and walnuts. Enjoy it served warm or cold.

1. Preheat the oven to 180°C/Fan 160°C/Gas 4. Line a 900g loaf tin with non-stick baking paper.

2. Place all the ingredients, apart from the nuts and chocolate chips, in a large bowl and blitz with a hand-held blender until combined. Stir in the nuts and chocolate chips.

3. Spoon the mixture into the prepared tin and bake in the oven for 50 minutes, or until a skewer inserted into the centre comes out clean.

4. Leave to cool in the tin, then turn out on to a wire rack.

5. Cut into 12 thin slices and store in an airtight container.

PER SERVING / 262 CALS / PROTEIN 8.4G / SUGAR 7.7G / FIBRE 0.5G / CARBS 11.7G

Ginger Roasted Rhubarb with Nut Crumble

SERVES **4** | **PREP** **10** mins | **COOK** **15–20** mins

350g rhubarb, cut at an
    angle into 3cm slices
1 tbsp coconut oil or
    butter, melted
1 ball of stem ginger in syrup,
    drained and finely chopped
2 tbsp full-fat crème fraîche,
    or dairy-free equivalent,
    to serve

For the Nut Crumble
40g walnuts,
    finely chopped
4 soft pitted dates,
    finely chopped
20g ground almonds
1 tbsp coconut oil

This is so good you might be tempted to lick the dish. The rhubarb and ginger caramelise and char slightly. Perfect served with a dollop of crème fraîche. It delivers a good dose of fibre as well.

1. Preheat the oven to 190°C/Fan 170°C/Gas 5. Line two baking trays with non-stick baking paper.

2. Spread the rhubarb on a prepared tray. Toss with the coconut oil or butter and scatter the stem ginger over the top. Bake in the oven for 15–20 minutes, or until soft and sticky.

3. Meanwhile, place the walnuts, dates, ground almonds and coconut oil in a bowl and rub the mixture between your fingers to make a crumble. Spread out on to a prepared tray and bake for 5–7 minutes, or until crisp and golden.

4. Serve the sticky rhubarb topped with the crumble and a dollop of crème fraîche.

———

PER SERVING / 221 CALS / PROTEIN 4.4G / SUGAR 5.5G / FIBRE 2.5G / CARBS 11.9G

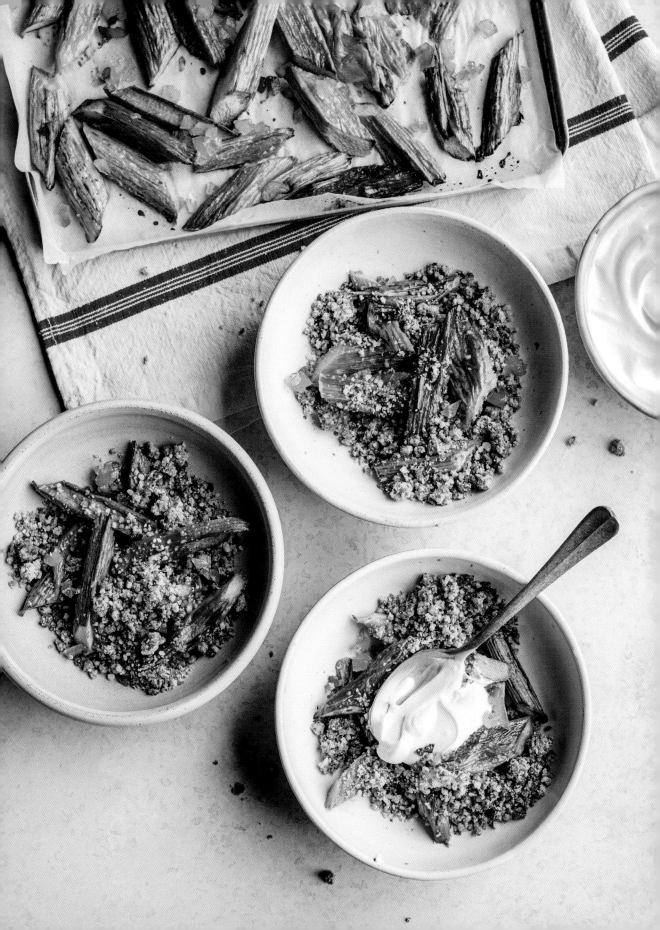

Spiced Sticky Toffee Apple Loaf

MAKES | **PREP** | **COOK**
8 | **20** mins | **30** mins

12 soft pitted dates,
    roughly chopped
70g coconut oil
80g wholegrain
    buckwheat flour
1 tsp bicarbonate of soda
½ tsp baking powder
2 tsp vanilla extract
2½ tsp ground cinnamon
1 tsp nutmeg (optional)
2 apples, cored and grated
    (120g prepared weight)
3 medium free-range eggs

COOK'S TIP
You can freeze this
by the slice and have
it ready to take out
from the freezer for
a quick treat.

This is a quirky take on a sticky toffee pudding,
using dates, cinnamon and fresh apple to create a
deliciously textured loaf. And to add to its credentials,
the buckwheat flour is high in fibre, as well as being
gluten free. Try it sliced when it is still warm or
toasted with a little bit of butter.

1. Heat the oven to 190°C/Fan 170°C/Gas 5.
Line a 500g loaf tin with non-stick baking paper.

2. Place the dates, coconut oil and 100ml of water
in a small saucepan, bring to the boil and simmer for
2 minutes. Blitz until smooth and set aside to cool.

3. Place the flour, bicarbonate of soda, baking powder,
vanilla extract, cinnamon, nutmeg, if using, grated
apples and eggs in a bowl and mix until combined.

4. Pour in the cooled date mixture and mix well.

5. Transfer to the prepared loaf tin and bake for
30 minutes, or until risen and a skewer inserted
in the centre comes out clean.

———

PER SERVING / 165 CALS / PROTEIN 3.9G / SUGAR 3.9G / FIBRE 0.6G / CARBS 12.1G

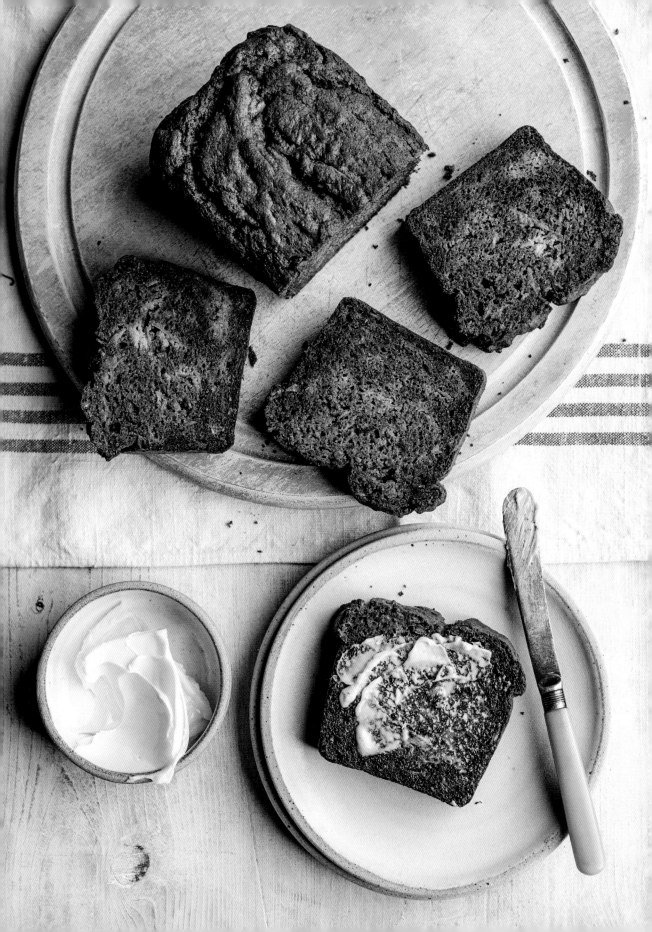

Chocolate Cake with Ginger Chocolate Ganache

SERVES	PREP	COOK
8	**20** mins	**35–40** mins

1 medium aubergine
   (eggplant), skin on, diced
50g dark chocolate (at least
   70%), broken into pieces
60g coconut oil
60g soft pitted dates, chopped
½ tsp salt
3 medium free-range eggs,
   beaten
1 tsp baking powder
80g ground almonds (or 100g
   gluten-free brown flour)

For the Chocolate Ganache
100ml full-fat coconut milk
70g dark chocolate (at least
   70%), broken into pieces
1 tsp coconut oil
2 balls of stem ginger in syrup,
   drained and finely chopped

Challenge anyone to identify the main ingredient of this fabulous creamy chocolate cake. It will keep everyone guessing.

1. Preheat the oven to 180°C/Fan 160°C/Gas 4. Grease and line a 20cm cake tin with non-stick baking paper.

2. Steam the aubergine (eggplant) for 15 minutes, or until soft, then place it in a bowl. While it is still hot, add the chocolate and coconut oil and stir until melted. Stir in the chopped dates, then blitz with a hand-held blender to obtain a smooth paste.

3. Add the salt, eggs, baking powder and ground almonds or gluten-free flour and blitz one more time. Spoon the mixture into the prepared tin and bake for 35–40 minutes, or until a skewer inserted into the centre comes out clean. Leave to cool in the tin for 10 minutes, then transfer to a wire rack.

4. Meanwhile, to make the ganache, place the coconut milk in a small saucepan over a medium heat and bring to the boil. Immediately remove from the heat and add the chocolate and coconut oil, and stir until melted. Add two thirds of the stem ginger and mix well.

5. Spread the ganache on top of the cakee, allowing it to dribble over the sides. Sprinkle with the remaining ginger and a pinch of salt and serve straight away, or refrigerate to allow the ganache to harden.

PER SERVING / 285 CALS / PROTEIN 6.8G / SUGAR 13.3G / FIBRE 1.9G / CARBS 14.2G

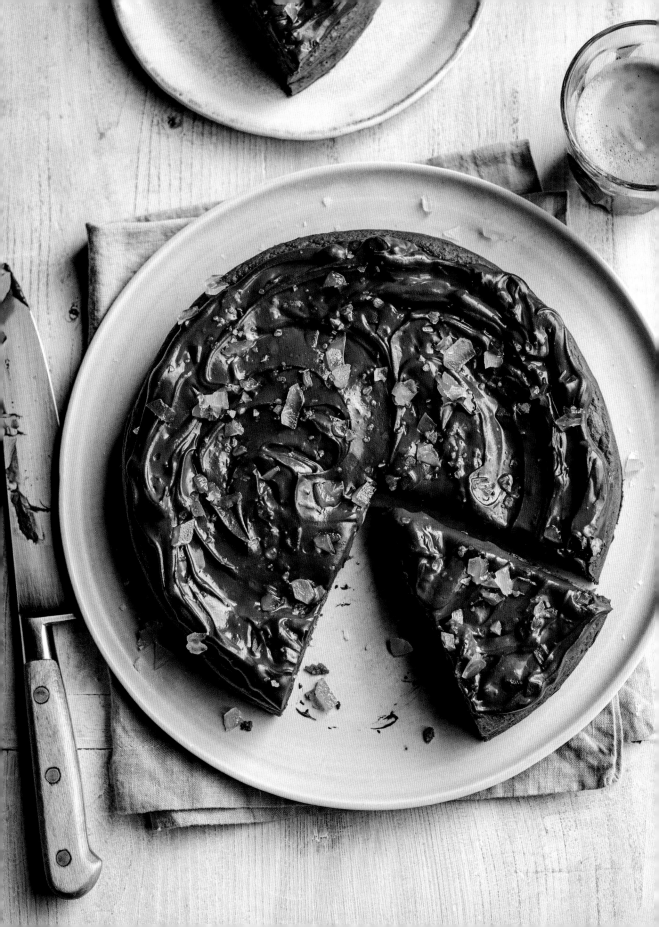

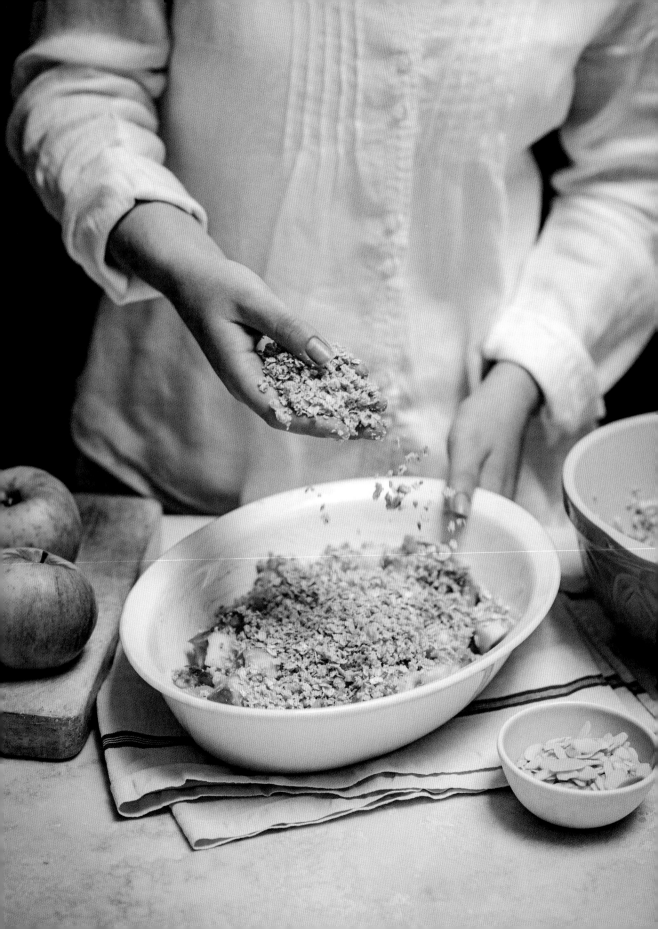

Desserts

Apple Crumble

SERVES	PREP	COOK
8	**15** mins	**40** mins

3–4 large cooking apples,
   cored and chopped into
   small cubes (about 600g
   prepared weight)
100g soft pitted dates, diced

For the Crumble
100g ground almonds
100g rolled oats
100g coconut oil, melted
50g flaked almonds

COOK'S TIP
The crumble mixture
freezes well. Top the
fruit with crumble
straight from the
freezer and bake.

Heart-warming comfort food without the sugar hit –
this lovely crumble is sweetened by dates and uses
rolled oats and ground almonds instead of flour, both
of which keep sugar spikes to a minimum. Nuts and
ground almonds provide healthy fats, proteins and fibre
that help to protect against heart disease and Type 2
diabetes. The crumble is delicious served with a
spoonful of Greek or non-dairy yoghurt.

1. Preheat the oven to 180°C/Fan 160°C/Gas 4. You will
need a roughly 30cm oval pie dish.

2. Place the apples and dates in the bottom of the pie dish.

3. Combine the ground almonds, oats and pinch of salt in
a medium bowl. Pour in the coconut oil and mix thoroughly
with a spatula. Spread over the fruit, then bake in the oven
for 20 minutes.

4. Remove the crumble from the oven, sprinkle the
flaked almonds on top and bake for a final 20 minutes,
until golden brown.

———

PER SERVING / 317 CALS / PROTEIN 6.5G / SUGAR 9.4G / FIBRE 2.4G / CARBS 23G

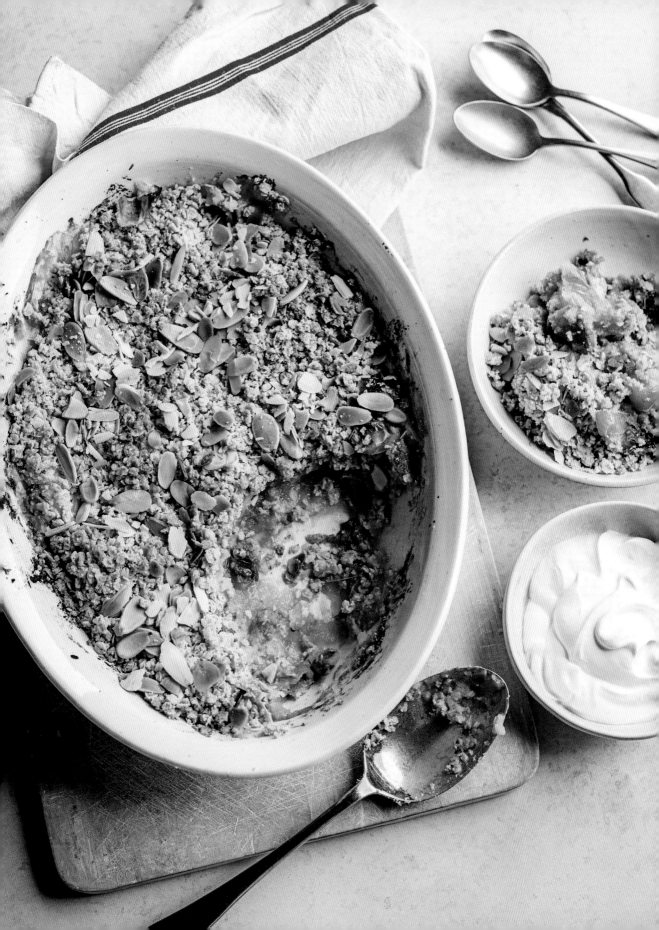

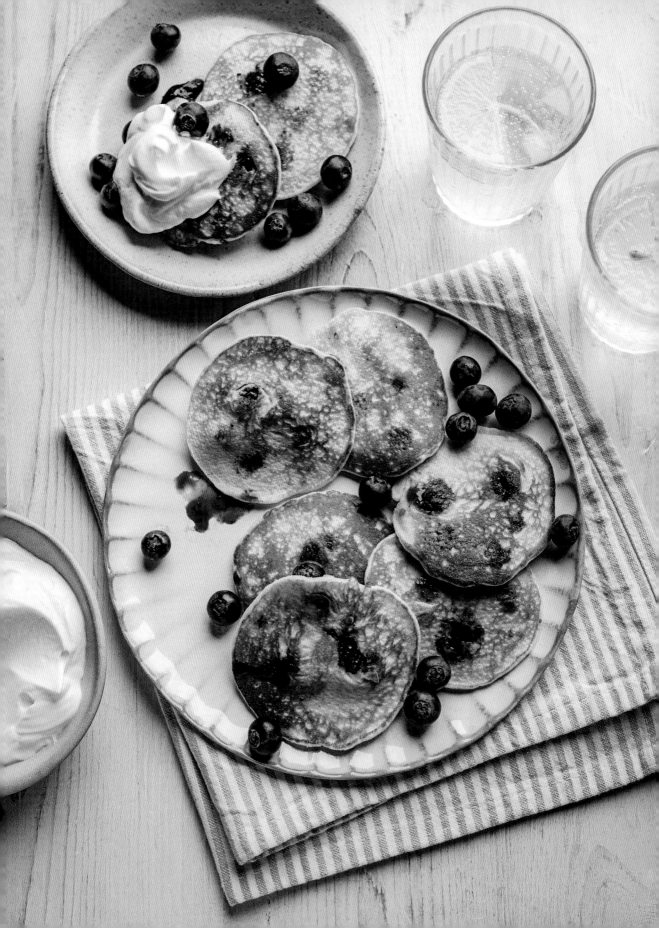

Blueberry Protein Pancakes

MAKES | **PREP** | **COOK**
8 | **5** mins | **8** mins

30g ground almonds
60g full-fat cream cheese,
   or dairy-free equivalent,
   softened
2 medium free-range eggs
½ tsp vanilla extract
80g blueberries, plus
   extra to decorate
15g butter (or coconut oil)

COOK'S TIP
The pancakes freeze well.
Store them with non-stick
baking paper between each
pancake so that it is easy to
remove one at a time. Thaw
them in the fridge and warm
gently in a medium oven
or for a short burst in the
microwave to serve.

Easy and delicious – these pancakes are lovely
served with yoghurt and more fresh blueberries.

1. Place the ground almonds, cream cheese, eggs
and vanilla extract in a medium bowl and mix with
an electric whisk until smooth. Stir in the blueberries.

2. Melt half the butter or coconut oil in a large non-stick
frying pan over a medium heat. Pour in four tablespoons of
batter to make 4 small pancakes. Cook for about 2 minutes,
or until golden, then flip and cook on the other side for the
same amount of time. Transfer to a plate and continue
with the rest of the butter and batter.

3. Serve the pancakes warm with extra blueberries
and full-fat Greek yoghurt, if you like.

———
PER SERVING / 79 CALS / PROTEIN 3.4G / SUGAR 1.3G / FIBRE 0.2G / CARBS 1.4G

Mixed Berry Fool

SERVES
2

PREP
5
mins

140g full-fat Greek yoghurt,
   or dairy-free equivalent
½ tsp vanilla extract
½ tsp honey
50g frozen mixed berries,
   defrosted

COOK'S TIP
If you only have fresh
berries, mash them before
adding to the yoghurt to
release some of the juice.

This elegant berry dessert is deceptively easy and
won't spike blood sugars due to the cushioning effect
of the full-fat Greek yoghurt. You could replace the
berries with any seasonal or tinned fruit, such as
apricots, cherries or diced mango.

1. Mix the yoghurt, vanilla extract and honey together
in a bowl.

2. Divide the yoghurt mixture between two small bowls.
Add the berries and stir gently to create a marbled effect.

PER SERVING / 107 CALS / PROTEIN 4.2G / SUGAR 5.9G / FIBRE 0.6G / CARBS 6.2G

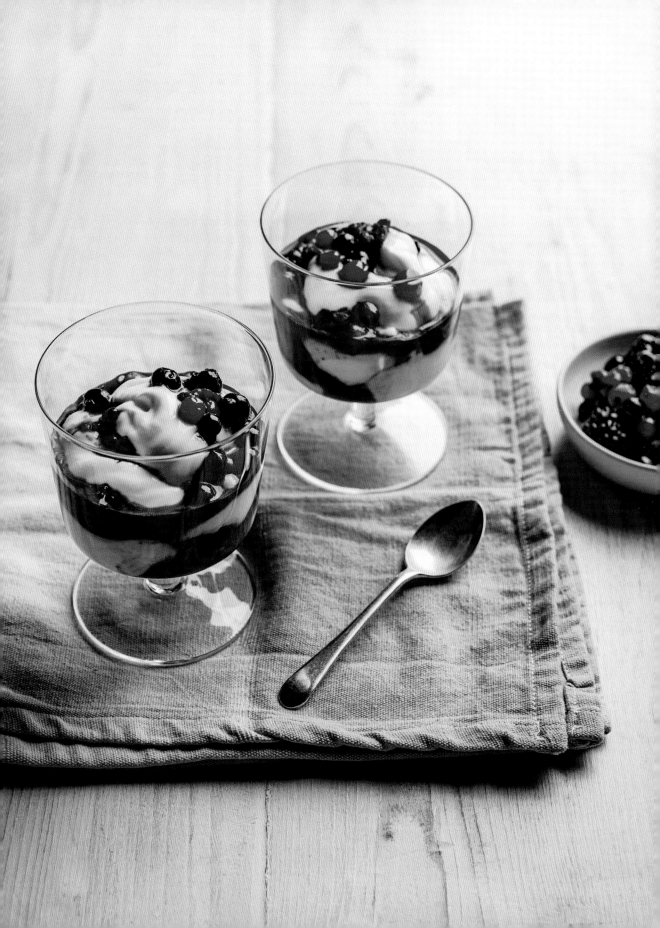

Almond and Plum Sponge Pudding

SERVES **8** | **PREP** **15** mins | **COOK** **30–40** mins

4 medium plums, stone
    removed and quartered
    (350g prepared weight)
125g coconut oil (or butter)
150g ground almonds
3 medium free-range eggs
2 tsp baking powder
100g soft pitted dates,
    roughly chopped
1 tsp almond extract (optional)

Almonds and plums are a classic combination, making an ideal autumn pudding to use up those abundant plums. This also works well with defrosted or even tinned plums (in juice, not syrup). Although we suggest removing the stones, we often decide to leave them in as its less fiddly to prepare – just remember to warn people to look out for them!

1. Preheat the oven to 190°C/Fan 170°C/Gas 5. Line a 20cm square baking dish with non-stick baking paper.

2. Lay two thirds of the plums in the prepared baking dish and set aside.

3. Place the coconut oil, ground almonds, eggs, baking powder, dates, almond extract, if using, and a pinch of salt in a food processor or blender and blitz to combine.

4. Pour the mixture over the plums, then press the remaining plums on to the surface for decoration. Bake in the centre of the oven for 30–40 minutes until turning golden on top.

5. Serve this with full-fat Greek yoghurt or Vanilla Cashew Cream (page 184).

PER SERVING / 325 CALS / PROTEIN 8.2G / SUGAR 8.2G / FIBRE 1.2G / CARBS 12G

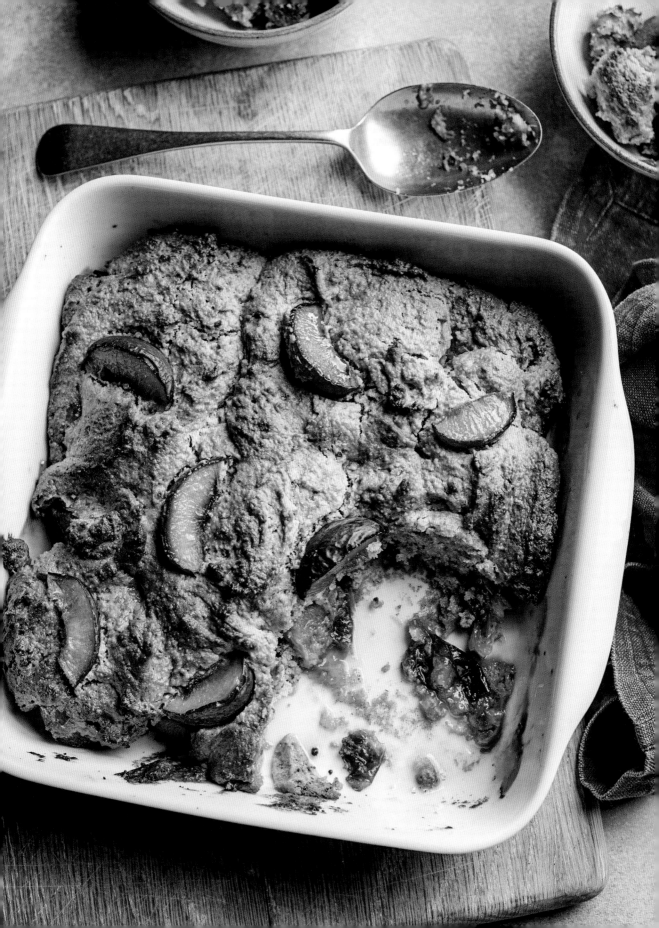

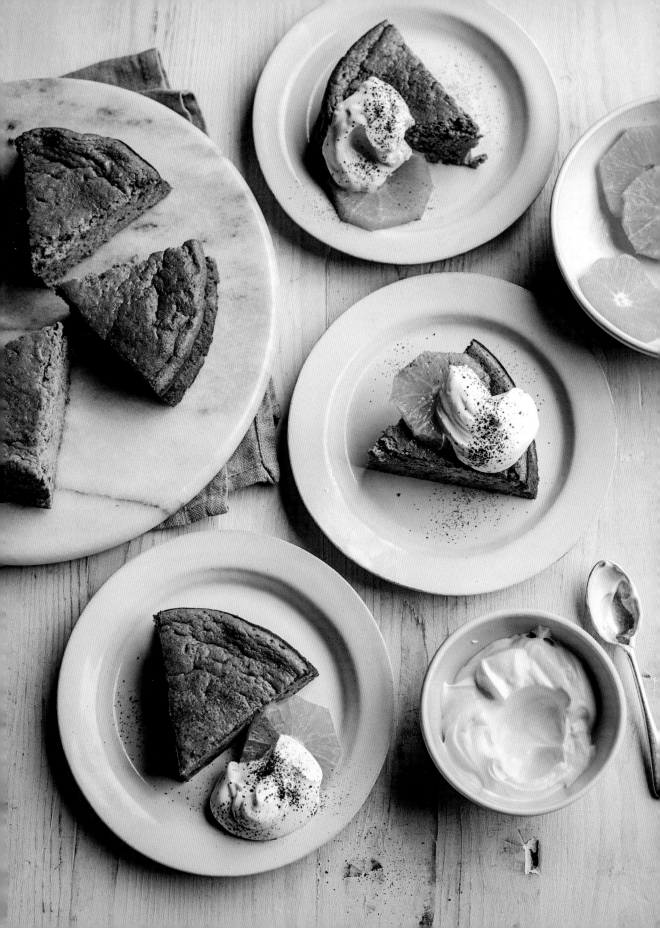

Coffee and Orange Ricotta Cheesecake

SERVES	PREP	COOK
6	**15** mins	**30–35** mins

½ tsp coconut oil, melted
5 soft pitted dates
250g soft ricotta cheese
1½ tbsp maple syrup
1 tbsp vanilla extract
Zest of 2 oranges plus
    2 tbsp juice
1 tbsp instant coffee
    (dissolved in 2 tbsp
    hot water)
25g wholegrain
    buckwheat flour
½ tsp baking powder
4 medium free-range
    eggs, separated

To Serve
1 orange, peeled and sliced
1 tbsp crème fraîche,
    per person

This luscious cheesecake is as light as a feather thanks to the ricotta and egg whites. Coffee and orange are a sophisticated and moreish flavour combination. This would make a great showstopper pudding.

1. Preheat the oven to 180°C/Fan 160°C/Gas 4. Line the base of an 18cm round springform tin with baking parchment. Use a pastry brush to grease the sides with the melted coconut oil. Set aside.

2. Place the dates, ricotta cheese, maple syrup, vanilla extract, orange zest and juice, and coffee in a food processor or blender and blitz until smooth. (If you are using a hand-held blender, make sure the mixture is as smooth as possible.)

3. Transfer the mixture to a bowl and add the flour, baking powder and egg yolks. Mix until thoroughly combined.

4. In a separate bowl, whisk the egg whites with a pinch of salt until stiff peaks form.

5. Fold a spoonful of the egg whites into the ricotta mixture, then add half the egg whites and fold in very gently. Finally fold in the remaining egg whites. Pour the mixture into the prepared tin and bake in the oven for 30–35 minutes, or until set. A skewer inserted into the centre should come out clean. Leave to cool in the tin.

6. Run a knife around the edges of the tin to loosen, then cut into 6 portions and serve with a slice of orange and a spoonful of crème fraîche.

PER SERVING / 211 CALS / PROTEIN 9.8G / SUGAR 6.1G / FIBRE 0.3G / CARBS 10G

Sourdough Bread and Butter Pudding

SERVES	PREP	COOK
4	**20** mins	**35–40** mins

200ml full-fat coconut milk
2 medium free-range eggs
1 tsp ground nutmeg
1 ball of stem ginger in syrup,
    drained and finely chopped
35g raisins
2 slices of brown or rye
    sourdough bread (about
    100g), sliced into 2cm cubes
20g shelled pistachios,
    roughly chopped

COOK'S TIP
You can freeze the
assembled but unbaked
pudding. Just thaw in
the fridge for 24 hours
before baking.

This classic homely dessert is made using sourdough bread and spices, which are transformed into a rich and creamy baked pudding with a golden brown, lightly crisped top layer.

1. Preheat the oven to 200°C/Fan 180°C/Gas 6.

2. Place the coconut milk, eggs, nutmeg, stem ginger and raisins in a bowl and mix well. Stir in the bread, then transfer to a 18cm round baking dish and set aside for 10 minutes to allow the bread to soak up the liquid.

3. Bake in the oven for 35–40 minutes, until the custard is set and the bread is golden brown and crisp on the surface.

4. Decorate with the pistachios to serve.

PER SERVING / 234 CALS / PROTEIN 7.9G / SUGAR 8.3G / FIBRE 1.7G / CARBS 18.3G

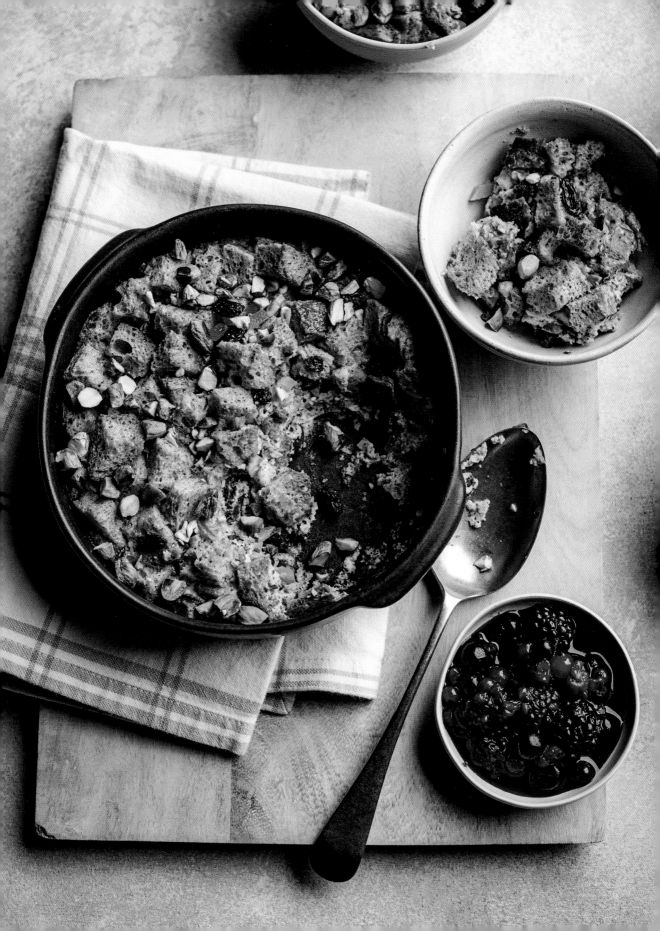

Cherry Chocolate Layer Dessert

SERVES	PREP	SET
4	**10** mins	**20** mins

1 × 425g tin of cherries, drained
   and roughly chopped
1 tbsp chia seeds
400g full-fat Greek yoghurt,
   or dairy-free equivalent
1 tsp vanilla extract
80g dark chocolate
   (at least 70%), grated
2 tbsp toasted flaked almonds

COOK'S TIP
If you're not eating these straight away, don't top with the almonds. Cover the desserts and they will keep in the fridge for a couple of days. Top with the flaked almonds just before serving.

Deceptively simple, this is a dreamy, creamy cherry dessert. Use a good-quality, full-fat live Greek yoghurt, or you could use half crème fraîche and half yoghurt, to make it even creamier.

1. Tip the cherries into a bowl and squash them with a fork. Stir in the chia seeds and leave to stand for 20 minutes.

2. Meanwhile, combine the yoghurt, vanilla extract and half the grated chocolate in a separate bowl.

3. Layer the cherries and yoghurt into four 250ml glass tumblers. Decorate with the rest of the grated chocolate and top with flaked almonds to serve.

PER SERVING / 322 CALS / PROTEIN 8.5G / SUGAR 25.7G / FIBRE 2.5G / CARBS 27.9G

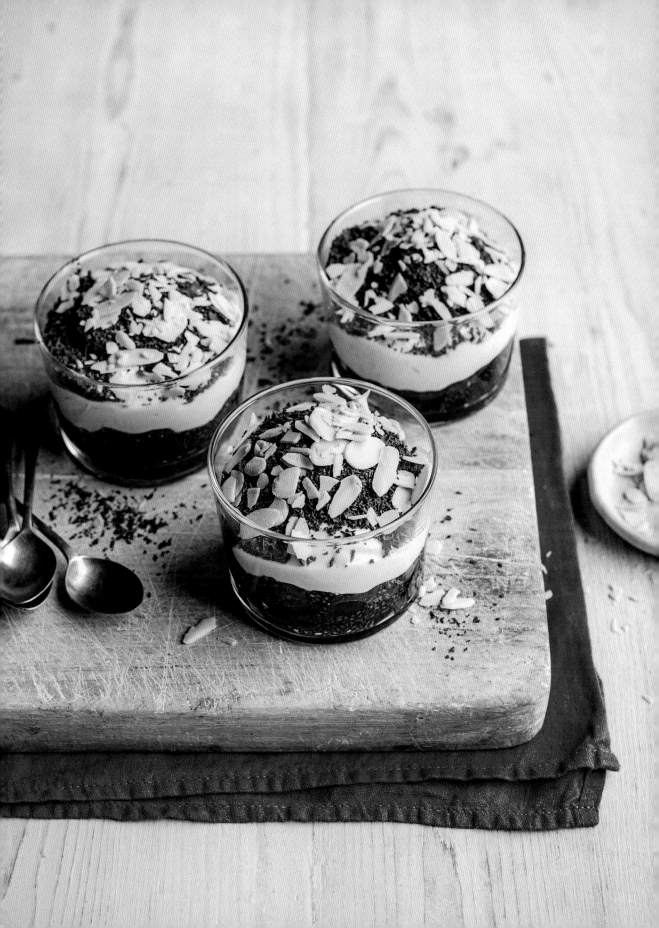

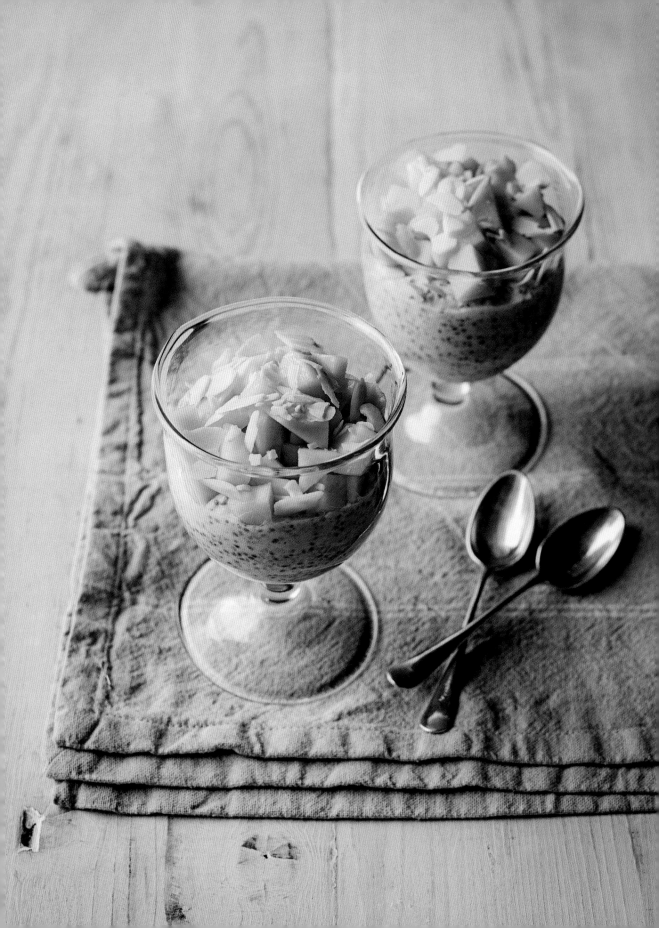

Mango and Lime Chia Pots

SERVES	PREP	SET
2	**5**	**30**
	mins	mins

30g chia seeds
100g full-fat Greek yoghurt
120ml full-fat milk
1 tsp vanilla extract
Zest of ½ lime
100g mango (roughly 1
    small mango), peeled
    and roughly chopped
1 tbsp flaked almonds

This luxurious and zingy mango recipe serves two, but the pots will keep for a few days in the fridge, making it a good dessert to prepare ahead. I am a big fan of chia seeds as they have interesting properties. An unassuming little seed, it produces a flavourless gel when soaked in water, making the pudding thicker and creamier. It also packs a punch when it comes to its impressive nutritional credentials, as it is high in protein, fibre and much-needed omega-3.

1. Place the chia seeds, yoghurt, milk, vanilla extract, lime zest and half the mango in a medium bowl and blitz for about 30 seconds with a hand-held blender. You want to retain some of the texture of the chia seeds.

2. Divide between two glasses and scatter the remaining mango on top.

3. Leave to set in the fridge for about 30 minutes. Top with the flaked almonds just before serving.

PER SERVING / 255 CALS / PROTEIN 11.1G / SUGAR 11.3G / FIBRE 7.4G / CARBS 18.3G

VEGAN | GLUTEN FREE | NUT FREE | DAIRY FREE

Chocolate Coconut Pudding with Pear

MAKES **4**

PREP **10** mins

SET **1** hour

4 soft pitted dates,
    roughly chopped
160ml coconut cream
½ tsp vanilla extract
75g dark chocolate (at least
    70%), broken into pieces
2 small pears

COOK'S TIP
Coconut or full-fat Greek yoghurt would make a nice addition to this dessert, allow ½ tablespoon per person. You could serve this with 50g raspberries per person instead of the pears, if you prefer.

A rich and creamy mousse with a delicate fruity tang. This is a perfect indulgence to round off a meal.

1. Place the dates, coconut cream and vanilla extract in a small saucepan over a medium heat. Bring to the boil and simmer for 30 seconds.

2. Remove from the heat, add the chocolate and a pinch of salt and stir until melted.

3. Blitz the mixture with a hand-held blender until smooth. Divide between four small glasses and refrigerate for 1 hour until set.

4. Meanwhile, core and slice the pears (you don't want to do this too much in advance or the fruit will brown). Divide the slices between the puddings to serve.

PER SERVING / 224 CALS / PROTEIN 2.2G / SUGAR 19.2G / FIBRE 2G / CARBS 22.2G

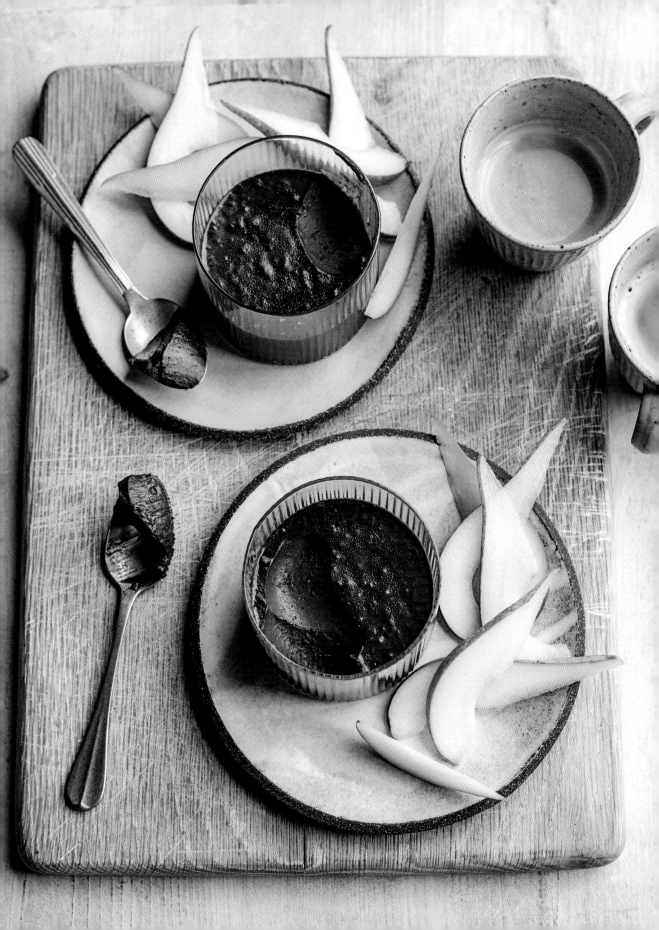

Rustic Filo Plum Tart

SERVES **4** | **PREP** **15** mins | **COOK** **15–20** mins

1 sheet filo pastry, halved
1 tbsp olive oil
1 tbsp vanilla extract
2 tbsp ground almonds
2 large plums, halved, stone
   removed and thinly sliced
   (200g prepared weight)
1 tbsp honey

The joy of filo pastry is that the delicate thin layers give a taste of pastry indulgence without the sugar-spiking effect of thicker pastry. This is a serious treat, yet it's easy to make. Heating the baking tray in the oven first helps the pastry to crisp on the base.

1. Preheat the oven to 200°C/Fan 180°C/Gas 6. Place a baking tray in the oven to get hot.

2. Lay a piece of non-stick baking paper the same size as the baking tray on a flat surface.

3. Brush each half of filo pastry with olive oil, then layer one on top of the other on the non-stick baking paper.

4. Mix the vanilla extract and ground almonds together to form a crumbly paste. Spread this on the pastry, leaving a 2.5cm border around the edge.

5. Arrange the sliced plums on top of the almond paste in a single layer. Drizzle the honey all over. Fold the edges of the pastry over the plums, creating a square-shaped tart with the plums exposed in the centre.

6. Remove the hot baking tray from the oven and carefully slide the tart and its non-stick baking paper on to the hot tray. Bake in the oven for 15–20 minutes, or until the edges are golden and crisp.

7. Slice in four and serve immediately with full-fat Greek yoghurt, if you like.

PER SERVING / 140 CALS / PROTEIN 3.1G / SUGAR 8.4G / FIBRE 1.4G / CARBS 14.6G

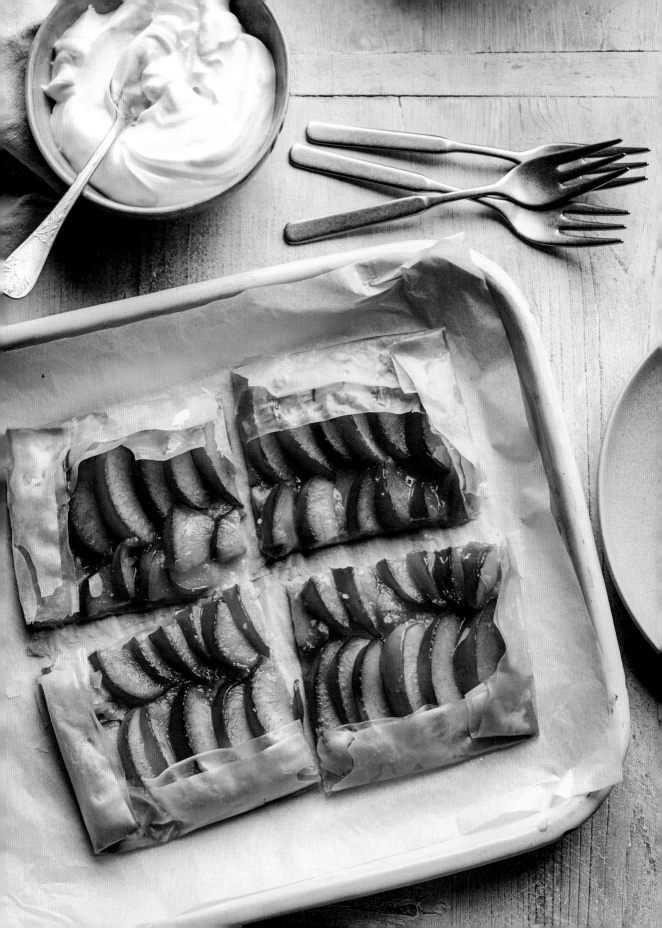

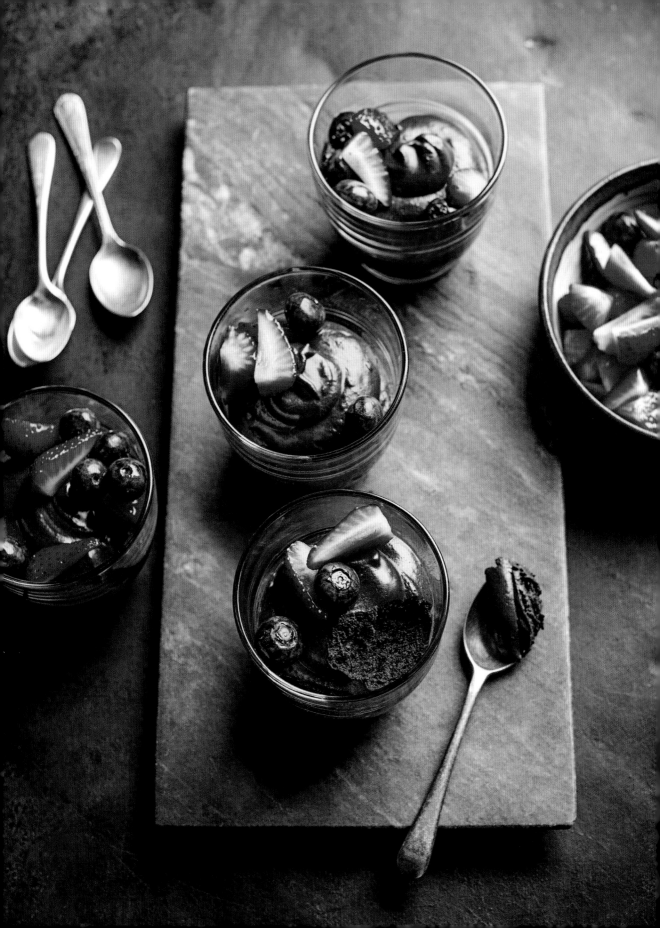

GLUTEN FREE NUT FREE DAIRY FREE

Three-Ingredient Chocolate Mousse

SERVES | PREP | SET
4 | **10** mins | **2** hours

125g dark chocolate (at least 70%), broken into pieces
1 tsp coconut oil
4 medium free-range egg whites

A surprisingly simple yet indulgent chocolate mousse.

1. Place the chocolate and coconut oil in a heatproof bowl over a saucepan of simmering water, making sure the bowl does not touch the water, and stir until melted. Remove from the heat and leave to cool for about 5 minutes.

2. Place the egg whites in a separate clean bowl with a pinch of salt and use an electric whisk to achieve stiff peaks.

3. When the chocolate has cooled, add a quarter of the egg whites to the chocolate and use the electric whisk to beat the egg whites in. This will stop the chocolate from seizing up. Now fold in the remaining egg whites with a spatula or metal spoon, until incorporated and the mousse is aerated and light.

4. Divide between four small glasses and refrigerate for about 2 hours, until set. Serve with berries, if you like.

———

PER SERVING / 183 CALS / PROTEIN 5G / SUGAR 18.6G / FIBRE 1G / CARBS 18.9G

Scorched Chilli Pineapple

SERVES	PREP	COOK
2	**10** mins	**4** mins

1 × 435g tin pineapple
(ideally stored in fruit
juice), drained and
chopped into 1–2cm pieces
¼–½ tsp chilli flakes
Handful of toasted nuts, such
as shelled pistachios, flaked
almonds or crushed walnuts
3–4 mint leaves, finely chopped
2 tbsp full-fat crème fraîche,
Greek yoghurt, or dairy-free
equivalent

Those of you who were around in the '70s might be delighted to try this old favourite with a chilli twist. Anyone younger will find intriguing bursts of sweet, juicy, tangy pineapple with a hint of chilli to cut through the sweetness. Pineapple also has a surprising range of health benefits, including containing antioxidants, vitamin C and fibre.

1. Place the pineapple on some kitchen roll to remove any remaining liquid.

2. Heat a griddle or frying pan until hot. Spread the pineapple pieces over the hot griddle, then scatter with the chilli flakes and a tiny pinch of salt. Lightly scorch the fruit for 4 minutes, turning halfway through.

3. Divide the slightly browned pineapple between two small plates, and top with the nuts and mint to decorate. Serve with a tablespoon of crème fraîche or full-fat Greek yoghurt alongside.

PER SERVING / 170 CALS / PROTEIN 2.8G / SUGAR 15.4G / FIBRE 0.9G / CARBS 15.4G

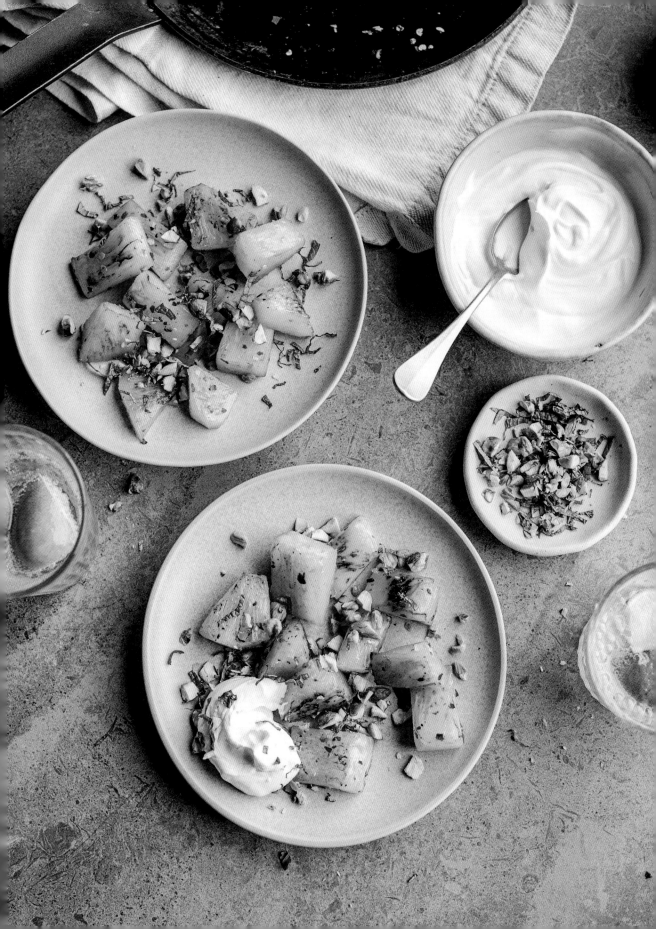

Coconut Quinoa Pudding

SERVES	PREP	COOK
4	**10** mins	**10–15** mins

1 × 400ml tin full-fat
   coconut milk
150g silken tofu
250g pre-cooked quinoa
1 tbsp chia seeds
1 tsp vanilla extract
1 tsp ground cardamom
   (or ground cinnamon)
1½ tbsp maple syrup
1 lime, cut into quarters
80g fresh berries, such as
   raspberries, strawberries
   or blueberries

COOK'S TIP
To cook 250g quinoa from
scratch, place 150g quinoa
in a small saucepan with
300ml water. Bring to a
simmer and cook with the
lid on for 7–10 minutes,
until the water is absorbed.
Remove from the heat and
leave covered for 5 minutes,
then fluff up to serve.

An ideal way to use up leftover quinoa, this is creamy,
nutty and exotic. This is best topped with fresh fruit
and a generous squeeze of lime.

1. Place the coconut milk and tofu in a jug and blitz
with a hand-held blender until smooth. Place in a
medium-sized non-stick saucepan with a pinch of
salt and all the remaining ingredients, except the
lime and berries, and bring to a simmer.

2. Continue to simmer over a low heat, stirring
occasionally, for 10–15 minutes, until the consistency
is loose and creamy.

3. Divide the pudding between four bowls and serve
with a wedge of lime squeezed over the top along with
some berries.

_____

PER SERVING / 329 CALS / PROTEIN 7.5G / SUGAR 8.7G / FIBRE 5.2G / CARBS 30.9G

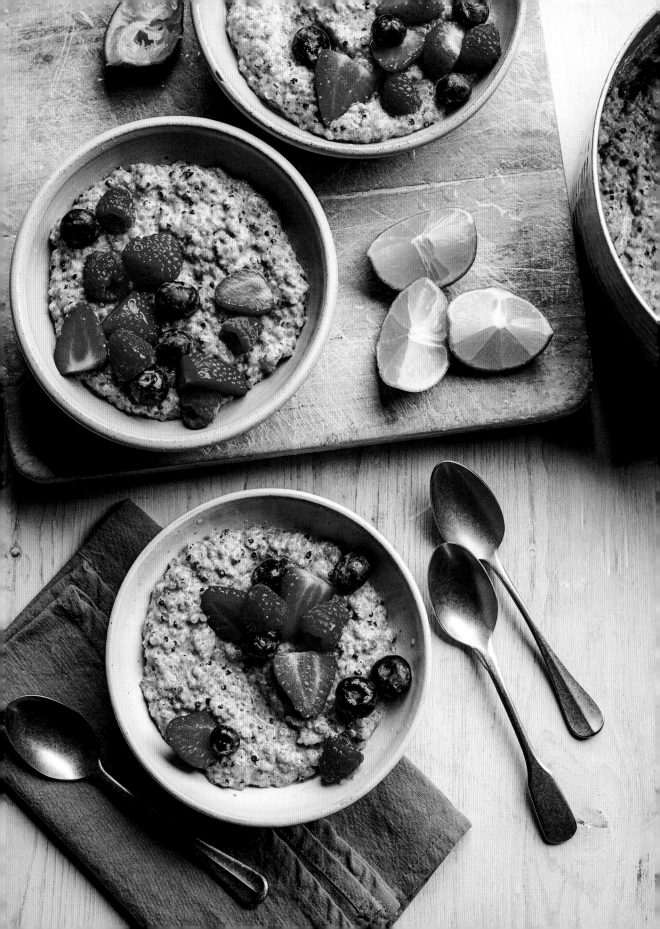

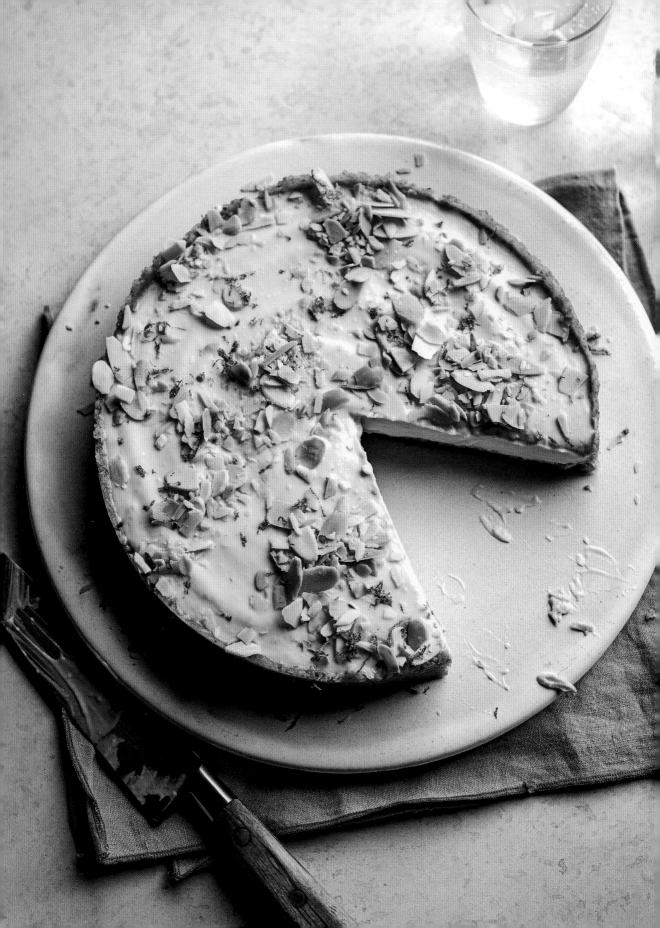

Avocado Lime Tart

SERVES **6** | **PREP** **20** mins | **SET** **2** hours

80g soft pitted dates
130g walnuts
2 tbsp coconut oil, melted
2 medium ripe avocados,
   peeled and stone removed
Zest and juice of 2 limes
½ × 400ml tin full-fat
   coconut milk
2 balls of stem ginger in syrup,
   drained and finely chopped
20g flaked almonds, toasted

COOK'S TIP
The tart will keep
for 2 days in the fridge.

There is something special about tucking into a tart, but if you don't have time for the base, you can just enjoy the delicious green mousse on its own. It sets beautifully in glasses, making it a refreshing and light dessert. Halve the recipe to make a mousse for two.

1. Line a 20cm round loose-bottomed cake tin with non-stick baking paper.

2. Place the dates and walnuts in a food processor or blender and blitz until finely chopped. Add the melted coconut oil and blitz again until the mixture is clumping together.

3. Tip the nutty mixture into the prepared tin and use the back of a spoon to press the mixture firmly into the base and sides. Set aside.

4. Place the avocados, lime zest and juice, coconut milk and stem ginger in a bowl and blitz with a hand-held blender until smooth. You could also make this in a food processor or blender.

5. Pour the avocado mixture into the tart case and smooth the surface. Refrigerate for at least 3 hours.

6. Decorate with the toasted almonds to serve.

_____

PER SERVING / 369 CALS / PROTEIN 6G / SUGAR 6.5G / FIBRE 3.4G / CARBS 7.9G

Chocolate Fruit Kebabs

SERVES	PREP	SET
4	**5** mins	**5–10** mins

100g dark chocolate (at least 70%), broken into pieces

1 large mango, peeled and cut into 12 chunks

½ melon, peeled and cut into 12 chunks

2 kiwis, peeled and each cut into 6 wedges

These gloriously colourful fruit kebabs can be assembled and enjoyed by children with a little supervision. They are higher in sugar than most other treats in this book, so aren't appropriate if you are on a 800–1000 fast day. However they are high in fibre – they have the second-highest fibre content per portion in the book! And eating a large variety of fruit and veg is wonderful for your gut, so these kebabs deserve their place among the other healthy treats.

1. Place the chocolate in a microwave-safe bowl and microwave for 30 seconds, then in bursts of 15 seconds, stirring each time, until melted.

2. Using four skewers, divide the fruit between the skewers, alternating the types of fruit as you go. There should be three pieces of each fruit on each skewer.

3. Place the skewers on non-stick baking paper, then spoon the melted chocolate over the top of the kebabs. Place in the fridge for 5–10 minutes to set.

PER SERVING / 214 CALS / PROTEIN 2.6G / SUGAR 31.3G / FIBRE 5.1G / CARBS 31.8G

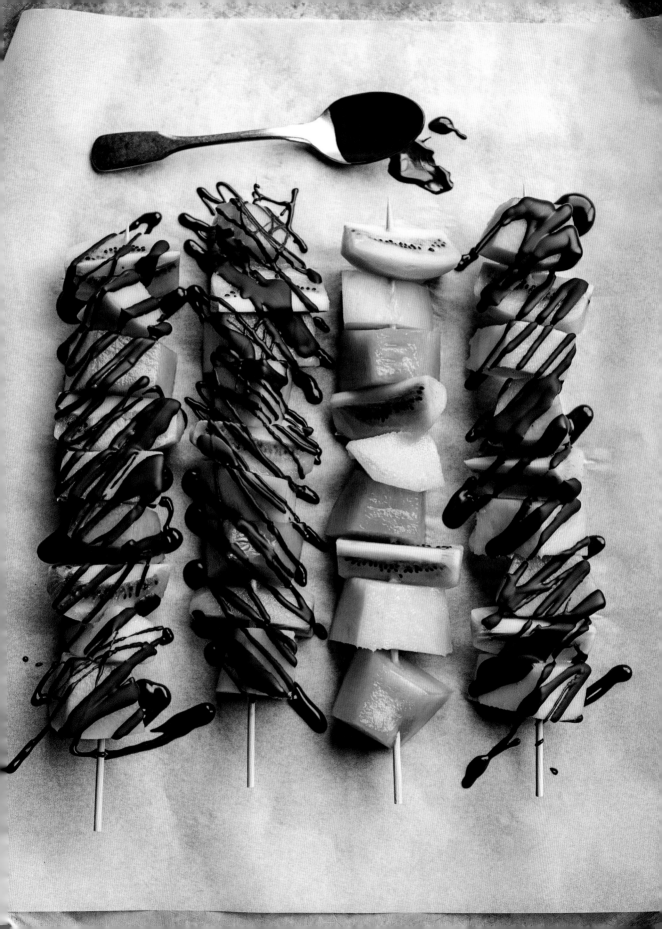

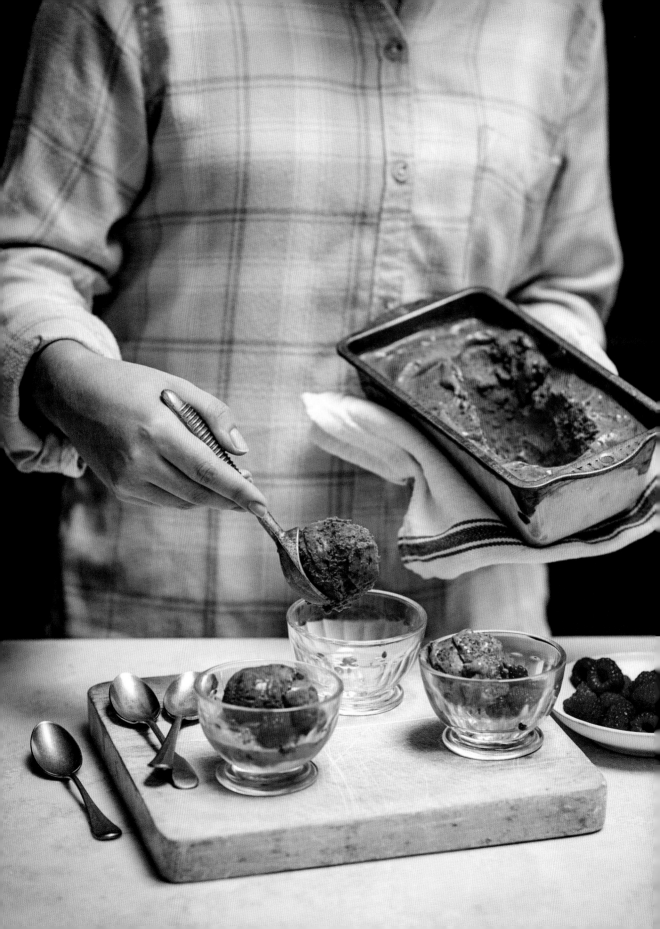

Frozen Treats

Creamy Coconut and Raspberry Ice Cream

SERVES	PREP	FREEZE
6	**5** mins	**4–5** hours

160ml coconut cream
200g frozen raspberries
1 medium banana, peeled
1 tsp vanilla extract
1 tbsp chia seeds

A velvety, fruity raspberry ice cream with a luxurious texture, enhanced by the creamy properties of the chia seeds. It's also surprisingly easy to make.

1. Place all ingredients in a bowl and blitz with a hand-held blender until smooth.

2. Transfer to a lidded container or individual pots and place in the freezer for 4–5 hours.

3. Remove from the freezer 5 minutes before serving to soften slightly.

PER SERVING / 92 CALS / PROTEIN 1.1G / SUGAR 6.3G / FIBRE 2G / CARBS 6.3G

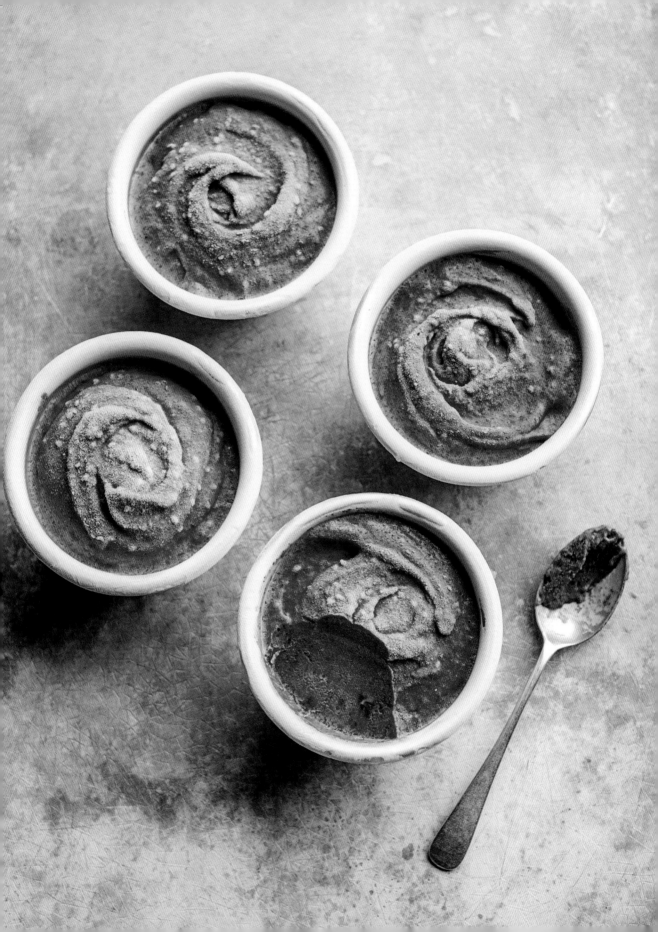

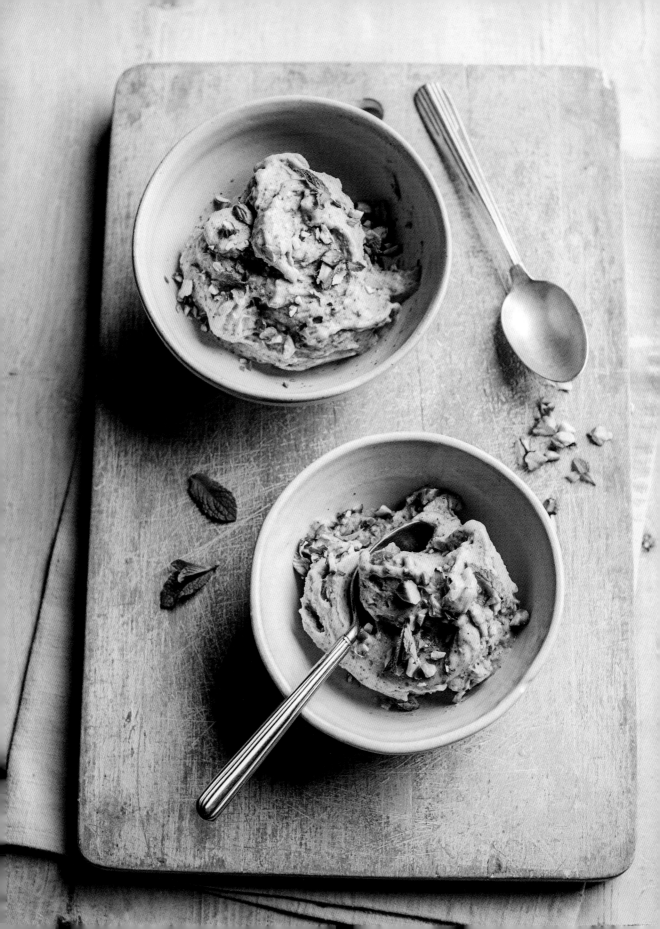

Banana Pistachio Ice Cream

SERVES | **PREP** | **FREEZE**
4 | **10** mins | **1** hour

2 small ripe bananas,
    peeled, sliced and frozen
50g shelled pistachios,
    chopped, plus another
    20g, to serve
5g fresh mint leaves,
    plus extra to serve

Simple, sweet and creamy with a nutty crunch,
a hint of mint and the bananas add probiotic fibre.
Surprisingly moreish!

1. Blitz all the ingredients together in a jug with
a hand-held blender until smooth. You could also
do this in a food processor or blender.

2. Serve at once with a few extra chopped nuts
and extra mint leaves sprinkled on top, or keep
in the freezer for another day.

PER SERVING / 106 CALS / PROTEIN 3.3XG / SUGAR 8.6G / FIBRE 0.7G / CARBS 9.8G

Astonishingly Simple Creamy Tangerine Sorbet

SERVES 2 | **PREP** 2 mins | **FREEZE** 1 hour

4 medium tangerines
   (mandarins), peeled
   and segments separated
2 tbsp full-fat Greek yoghurt,
   or dairy-free equivalent
A few chopped mint leaves,
   for decoration (optional)

An elegantly simple sorbet based on blitzing frozen tangerine (mandarin) segments. It's sweet and tart with a creamy orange flavour. Fun to make with the help of little ones – kids will love to eat it, too.

1. Put the tangerine (mandarin) pieces on a small tray or plate and place in the freezer for 1 hour at least.

2. Place the frozen segments in a food processor or blender with the yoghurt and blitz to make a creamy, tangy sorbet.

3. Share between two bowls and scatter over the mint, if using.

———

PER SERVING / 66 CALS / PROTEIN 1.8G / SUGAR 10G / FIBRE 1.4G / CARBS 5G

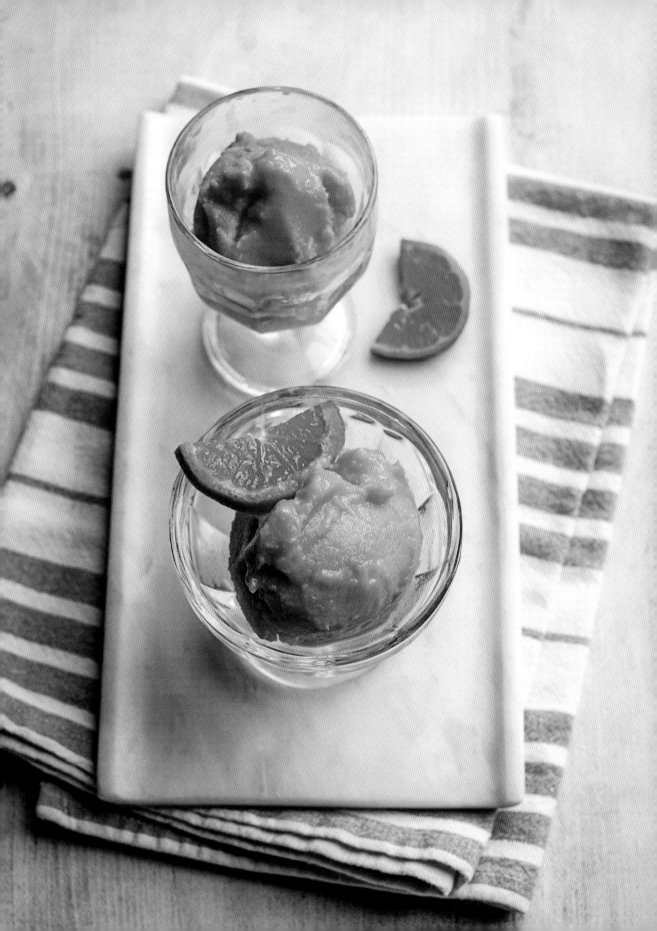

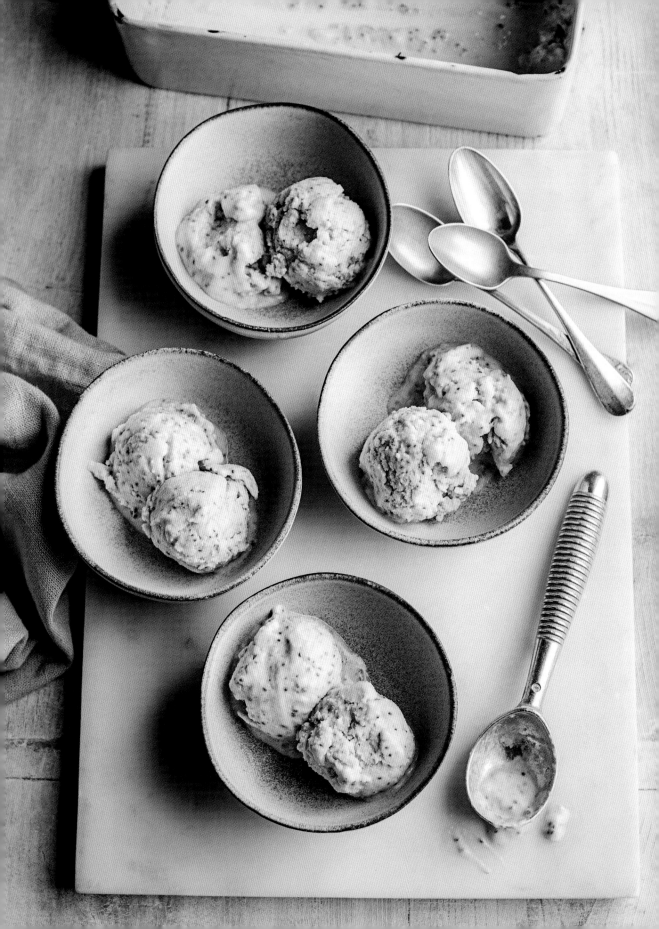

Ginger Frozen Yoghurt

SERVES **4**

PREP **15** mins

FREEZE **5** hours

2 balls of stem ginger in syrup, drained and finely chopped

1 tsp stem ginger syrup (from the jar)

150g full-fat Greek yoghurt, or dairy-free equivalent

1 medium ripe banana, peeled and mashed

1 tsp coconut oil

Cook's Tip

Adding chia seeds will increase the creaminess of this dessert and add some extra protein, too. If using, stir 1 teaspoon of chia seeds into the yoghurt mixture before freezing.

Tangy yoghurt is sweetened with ginger and banana for a wonderful frozen treat. Chia seeds increase the creaminess and add some extra protein, too.

1. Place all the ingredients, except the chia seeds, in a high-sided bowl or jug and blitz with a hand-held blender until smooth. Stir through the chia seeds.

2. Pour into a lidded plastic container and place in the freezer for about 5 hours.

_____

PER SERVING / 109 CALS / PROTEIN 2.4G / SUGAR 17.7G / FIBRE 0.5G / CARBS 14.5G

Cherry Swirl Almond Ice Cream

SERVES	PREP	FREEZE
4	**15** mins	**4–5** hours

200g silken tofu
1 tbsp coconut oil
60g full-fat Greek yoghurt,
   or dairy-free equivalent
1 tsp almond extract
2 dried apricots, chopped
100g frozen cherries
1 tbsp maple syrup

Top this ice cream with some toasted flaked almonds just before serving for extra texture.

1. Place the tofu, coconut oil, yoghurt, almond extract and apricots in a food processor or blender and blitz until smooth. Pour into a medium-sized plastic tub.

2. Rinse the blender, then add the frozen cherries and maple syrup. Blitz until completely smooth.

3. Swirl the cherry purée through the ice cream base, creating a marbled effect. Place in the freezer for 4–5 hours.

PER SERVING / 105 CALS / PROTEIN 4.5G / SUGAR 7.4G / FIBRE 0.5G / CARBS 8.4G

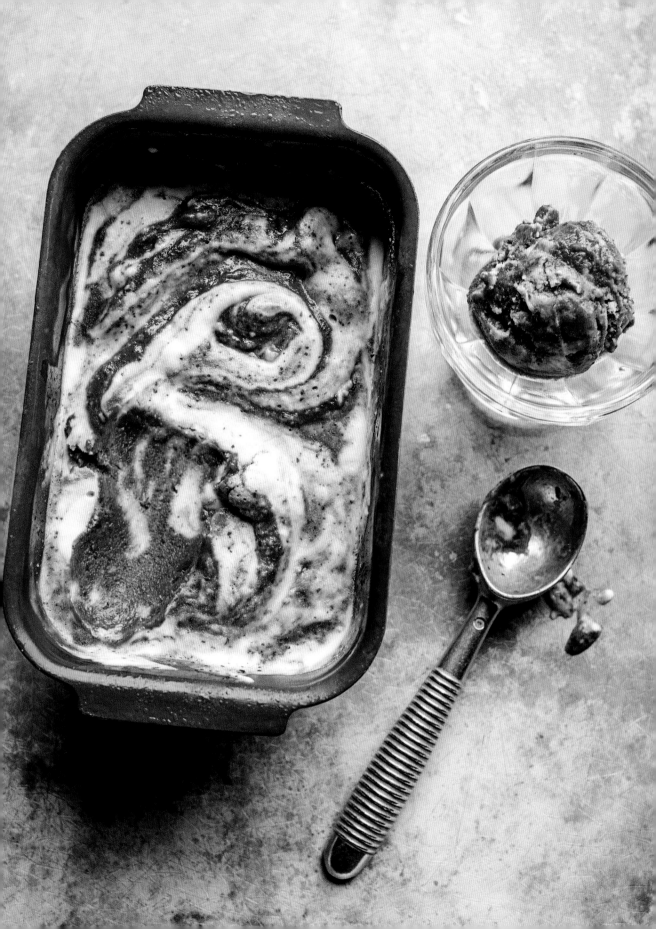

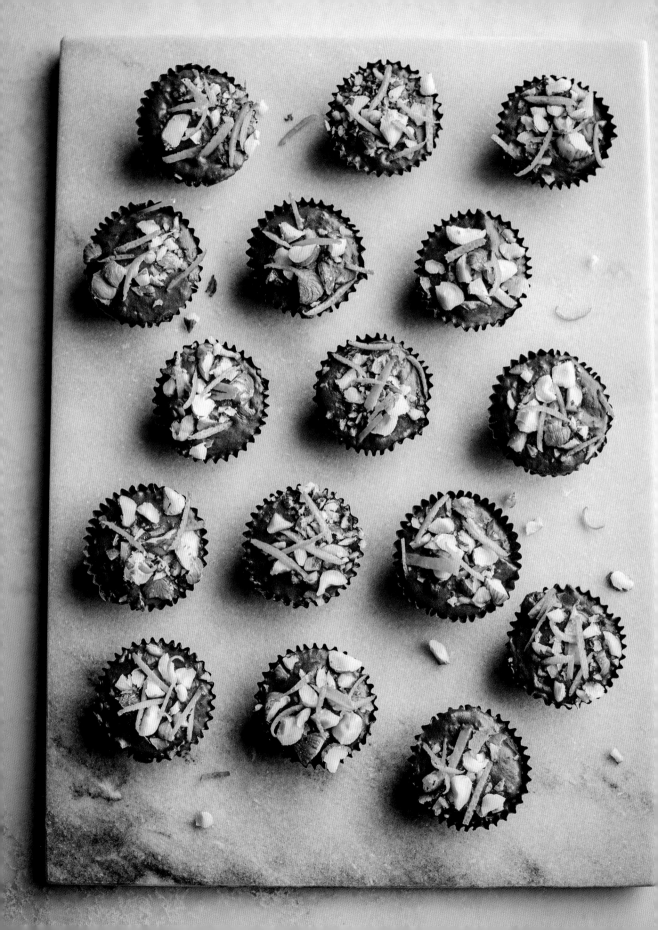

Frozen Chocolate Orange Cupcakes

MAKES
8

PREP
10
mins

FREEZE
30
mins

75g dark chocolate (at least 70%), broken into pieces

1 medium ripe banana, peeled and well mashed

Zest of ½ medium or large orange

Finely shredded peel of ½ medium or large orange

1 tbsp finely chopped toasted hazelnuts

These cute, little, melt-in-the-mouth frozen chocolate cupcakes deliver an almost truffle-like bite, yet only take 10 minutes to make and are ready to pull out of the freezer 30 minutes later. They store well in the freezer in a sealed container.

1. Line a mini cupcake trap with 8 mini cases.

2. Place the chocolate in a microwave-safe bowl and microwave for 30 seconds, then in bursts of 15 seconds, stirring each time, until melted.

3. Add the banana and orange zest to the melted chocolate and mix well.

4. Divide the mixture between the mini cupcake cases, then gently press a few pieces of shredded peel into the surface of each one and scatter with the hazelnuts for decoration.

5. Place the cupcake cases in the freezer and leave to set for at least 30 minutes.

6. Serve straight from the freezer.

PER SERVING / 75 CALS / PROTEIN 1G / SUGAR 8.8G / FIBRE 0.7G / CARBS 8.8G

Mango and Lime Sorbet

SERVES
2

PREP
10
mins

150g frozen mango chunks
Zest of 1 lime
65g coconut yoghurt
1 tsp honey

Mango and lime are a match made in heaven. This is super quick and easy to make, and tastes delicious.

1. Place all the ingredients in a food processor or blender and blitz until smooth.

2. Divide between two bowls and eat at once, or keep in the freezer until needed.

PER SERVING / 84 CALS / PROTEIN 0.7G / SUGAR 14.1G / FIBRE 2.7G / CARBS 15.4G

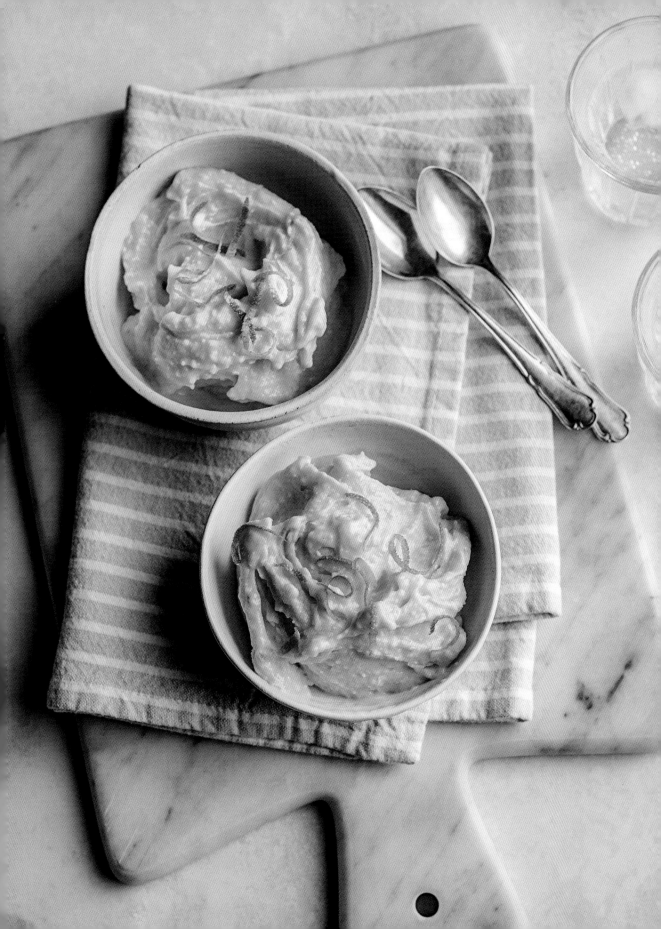

Strawberry and Cream Ice Pops

SERVES | **PREP** | **FREEZE**
4 | **5** mins | **4** hours

250g frozen strawberries
100g full-fat Greek yoghurt,
   or dairy-free equivalent
1 tbsp honey
1 tbsp chia seeds

This is a fantastic recipe for children (and adults!) as well as being a great way of using up overripe strawberries.

1. Place all the ingredients in a food processor or blender and blitz until smooth.

2. Pour into four ice-lolly moulds (each about 75ml) and freeze for 4 hours.

PER SERVING / 47 CALS / PROTEIN 1.6G / SUGAR 3.2G / FIBRE 1.4G / CARBS 3.3G

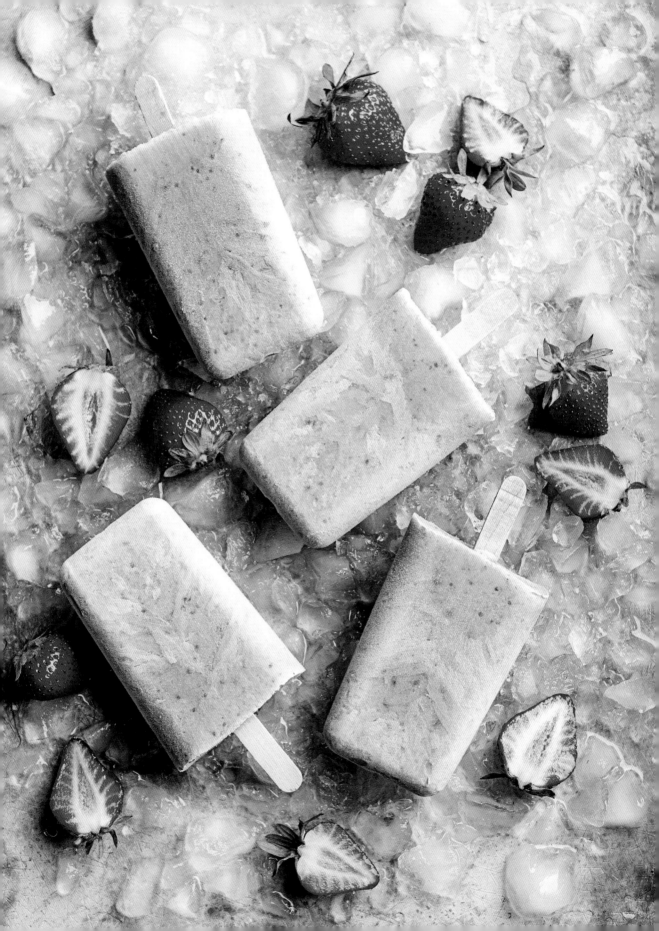

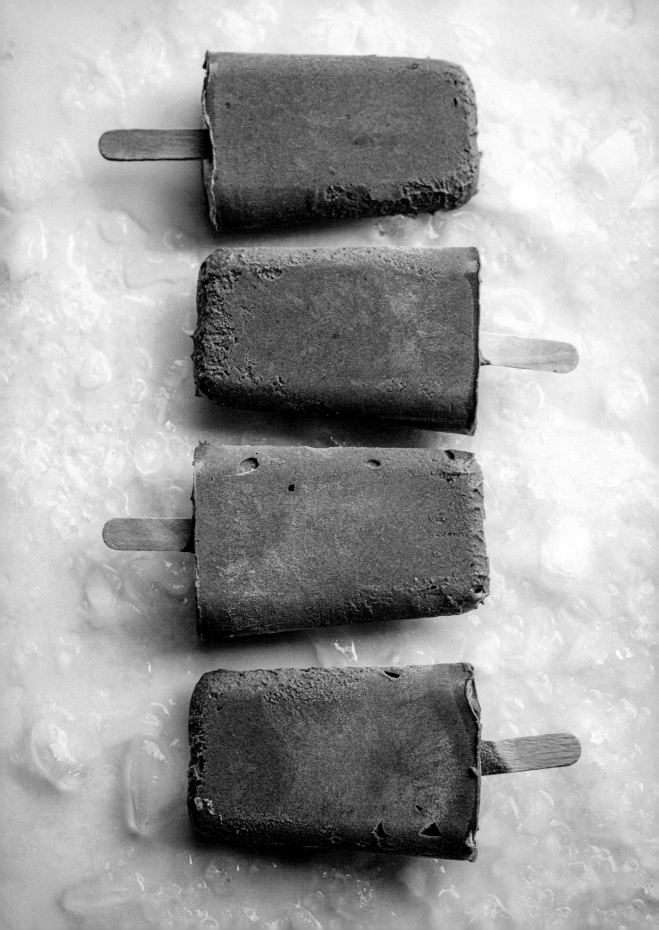

Avo-banana Chocolate Lollies

MAKES
4

PREP
10 mins

FREEZE
3–4 hours

1 medium ripe avocado,
   peeled and stone removed
25g unsweetened
   cocoa powder
1 large ripe banana
   (or 2 small), peeled
   and mashed
160ml coconut cream
1 tbsp vanilla extract
80g soft pitted dates,
   chopped (or date paste)
½ tsp flaky sea salt
½ tbsp balsamic vinegar
   (optional)

These have quite a grown-up flavour. I love them with the extra tang of balsamic vinegar, but you could leave this out.

1. Place all the ingredients in a food processor or blender and blitz until smooth.

2. Spoon it four ice-lolly moulds and freeze for 3–4 hours.

PER SERVING / 123 CALS / PROTEIN 2G / SUGAR 12.2G / FIBRE 3.1G / CARBS 14.1G

Chocolate Raspberry Nutty Bites

MAKES	PREP	FREEZE
14	**5** mins	**1** hour

1 × 180g bar dark chocolate
  (at least 70%)
14 fresh or frozen raspberries
14 tsp unsweetened crunchy
  peanut butter
25g cashew nuts,
  roughly chopped

You will need one or two
  ice-cube trays

An easy no-cook nutty indulgence. Raspberry and chocolate are made for one another. Using dark chocolate has numerous health benefits and it also tends to be less 'addictive' so if, like Michael, you are partial to milk chocolate, it's a good swap. I still have to hide any chocolate that's in the house, though!

1. Place the chocolate in a microwave-safe bowl and microwave for 30 seconds, then in bursts of 15 seconds, stirring each time, until melted.

2. Using 14 squares of the ice-cube tray(s), pour 1 teaspoon of melted chocolate into each square.

3. Top each one with 1 raspberry, 1 teaspoon of peanut butter, a final drizzle of of chocolate and 1 teaspoon of chopped cashews to finish.

4. Freeze for at least 1 hour, then pop the bites out of the tray(s). Store in the freezer and allow to defrost for 5 minutes before eating.

PER SERVING / 109 CALS / PROTEIN 2.4G / SUGAR 8.1G / FIBRE 1G / CARBS 9.6G

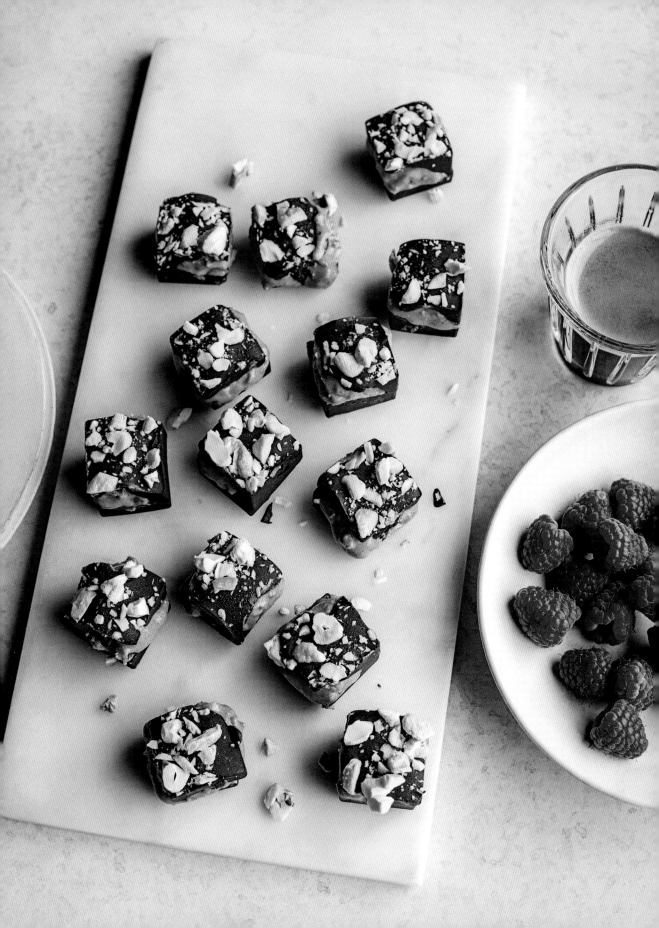

Peach and Mint Granita

SERVES	PREP	FREEZE
4	**10** mins	**3–4** hours

1 × 410g tin peaches (ideally
   stored in fruit juice), drained
A few sprigs of fresh mint,
   leaves picked and
   finely chopped
4 tbsp coconut yoghurt

COOK'S TIP
You may want to
allow 5–10 minutes
for the granita to
soften before serving.

Neither ice cream, nor sorbet, nor slushie, this makes
an elegant and interesting dessert. Zingy, crunchy
and beautifully cooling!

1. Place the peaches in a food processor or blender
and blitz until smooth. Stir in the chopped mint.

2. Pour into a lidded plastic container and place
in the freezer for 3–4 hours to set.

3. To serve, divide the yoghurt between four bowls
or glasses. Break up the granita with a fork and
divide between the bowls or glasses.

PER SERVING / 39 CALS / PROTEIN 0.5G / SUGAR 6.4G / FIBRE 0.7G / CARBS 7.1G

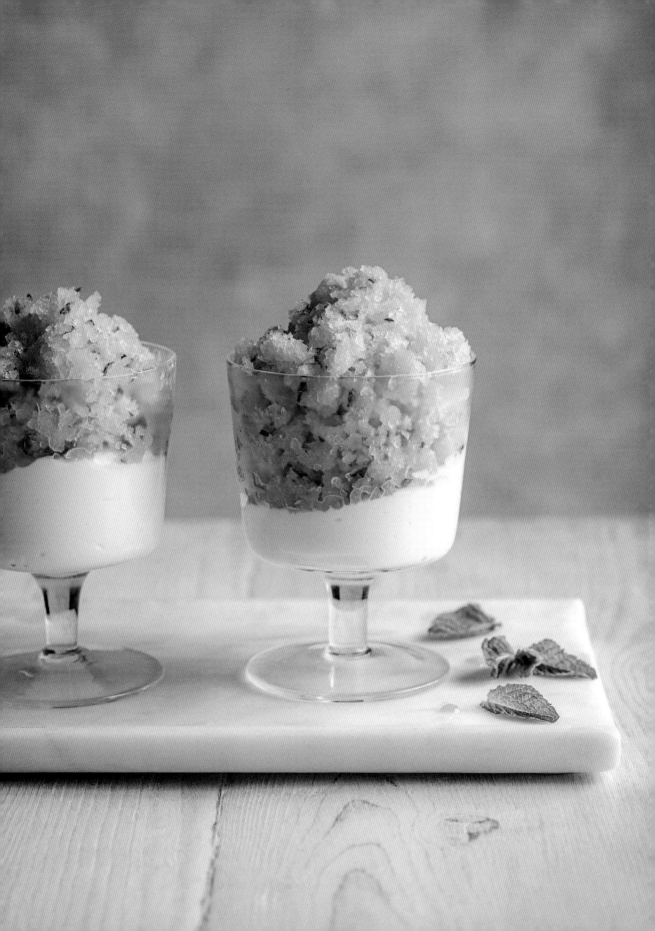

Smoothies

Smoothies make a quick and delicious meal or treat. The secret to making a healthy and nutritious smoothie is to make sure you include protein – whether tofu, yoghurt, full-fat milk, nuts or chia – and keep the sugar low by using berries, or other fruits that have a low sugar content. A smoothie is also a good way of adding more vegetables to your diet. The greater the variety of vegetables you eat each day, the better your gut health – so add handfuls of spinach, for example, or fresh herbs. Adding ice cubes or frozen fruit to the blender turns an ordinary smoothie into a frozen treat! It's worth remembering that blitzing only briefly, so you keep a bit of texture, actually increases the amount of fibre in the smoothie.

Kiwi, Pineapple and Spinach Smoothie

SERVES 2 | **PREP** 5 mins

1 kiwi, peeled
50g frozen pineapple
25g fresh spinach
15g cashew nuts
50g full-fat Greek yoghurt
    or dairy-free alternative
200g full-fat milk or
    dairy-free alternative
1 tsp honey
8 cubes of ice

This smoothie is deliciously refreshing and packed with goodness.

1. Place all the ingredients in a food processor or blender and blitz until smooth.

2. Serve immediately in two tall glasses.

———

PER SERVING / 185 CALS / PROTEIN 7.1G / SUGAR 14.5G / FIBRE 1.9G / CARBS 15.6G

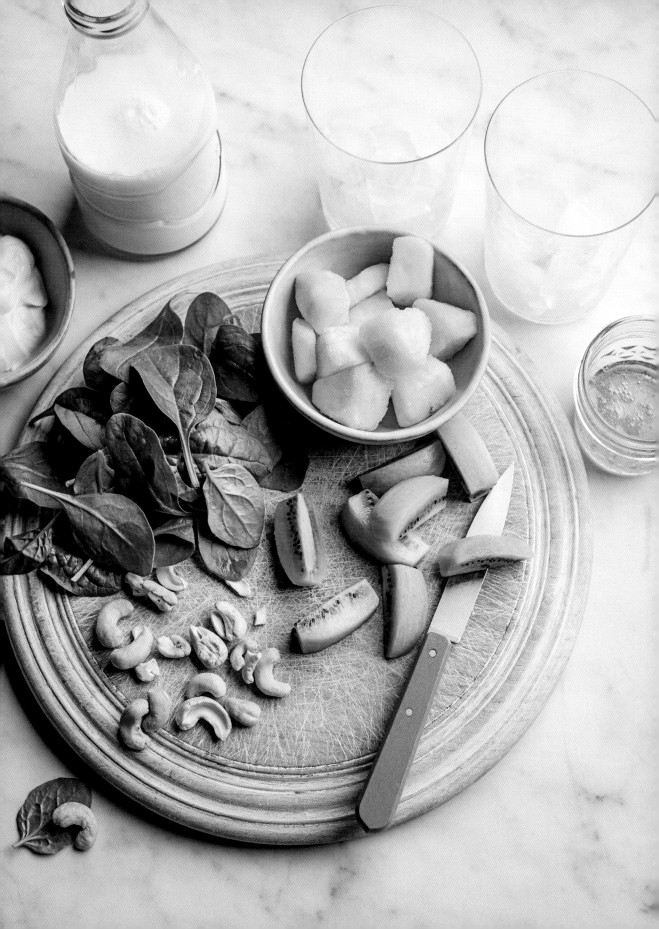

Tropical Fruit, Mint and Cucumber Cooler

SERVES **2** | **PREP** **5** mins

150g frozen tropical fruit mix
(such as papaya, mango
and pineapple)
50g cucumber
50g silken tofu
200ml full-fat milk or
dairy-free alternative
1 sprig of mint, leaves picked
Juice of 1 lime
1 tsp honey

A fresh and fruity, protein-rich smoothie, thanks to the added silken tofu.

1. Place all the ingredients in a food processor or blender and blitz until smooth.

2. Serve immediately in two tall glasses.

———

PER SERVING / 148 CALS / PROTEIN 7.3G / SUGAR 15.5G / FIBRE 2.2G / CARBS 16.1G

Banana and Almond Smoothie

SERVES **2** | **PREP** **5** mins

1 medium banana, peeled
150ml full-fat milk or
dairy-free alternative
1 tbsp almond butter
1 tsp maple syrup
1 tsp ground cinnamon
8 cubes of ice

The addition of ice makes this smoothie more like a slushie – it is cold and refreshing while also being filling.

1. Place all the ingredients in a food processor or blender and blitz until smooth.

2. Serve immediately in two tall glasses.

———

PER SERVING / 141 CALS / PROTEIN 4.5G / SUGAR 16.2G / FIBRE 0.7G / CARBS 16.2G

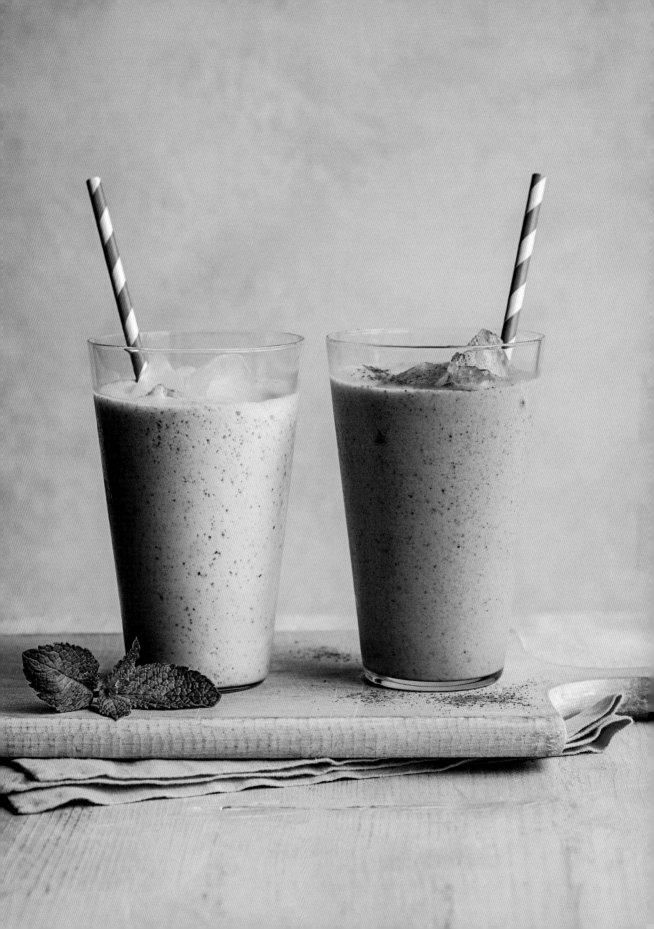

Frostings & Other Useful Recipes

Apricot and Lemon Cream Cheese Frosting

This is a delicious frosting which goes well with lots of different flavours. Try it with the Double Chocolate Cupcakes (page 54), or use it as an alternative frosting for the Chocolate Cake with Ginger Chocolate Ganache (page 122). It would good as a tart filling – make the cases as for the Cheat Custard Tarts (page 102) but fill them with this frosting instead.

Makes enough to cover 12 cupcakes or muffins

3 dried apricots
125g full-fat cream cheese
2 tbsp full-fat Greek yoghurt
1 tsp vanilla extract
Zest of 1/2 lemon

Place the apricots in a food processor and blitz until they are finely chopped.

Add the remaining ingredients and blitz again until combined.

Use immediately or transfer to an airtight container and keep in the fridge for 3–4 days.

PER SERVING / 341 CALS / PROTEIN 8.6G / SUGAR 12.5G / FIBRE 1.8G / CARBS 12.5G

Stem Ginger and Cream Cheese Frosting

This is a lovely, delicately flavoured frosting which will go well with lots of different flavours.

Makes enough to cover 12 cupcakes or muffins

125g full-fat cream cheese or mascarpone cheese
2 tbsp full-fat Greek yoghurt
1 1/2 tsp diced ginger in syrup

Place all the ingredients in a bowl and beat together until smooth.

Use immediately or transfer to an airtight container and keep in the fridge for 3–4 days.

PER SERVING / 330 CALS / PROTEIN 7.9G / SUGAR 10.9G / FIBRE 0.4G / CARBS 11.7G

Vanilla Cashew Cream

A wonderful alternative filling for the tart cases on page 102.

Makes enough for 4 portions

120g cashews, soaked in hot water for about 1 1/2 hours
1 tsp vanilla paste (or 2 tsp vanilla extract)
Juice of 1/2 small lemon
1/2 tbsp honey or maple syrup

Drain the cashews and place them in a bowl with the vanilla paste, lemon juice, honey, a pinch of salt and 175ml fresh cold water. Use a hand-held blender to blitz the nuts until you have a smooth mixture that resembles pouring cream. This could take 4–5 minutes. Add a little more water, if necessary, a tablespoon at a time, until you reach the right consistency. You could also do this in a food processor.

Transfer to an airtight container and keep in the fridge for up to 3 days.

PER SERVING / 186 CALS / PROTEIN 6.3G / SUGAR 3.2G / FIBRE 1.3G / CARBS 7.1G

Conversion Tables

Weight

5g	$\frac{1}{8}$oz
10g	$\frac{1}{4}$oz
15g	$\frac{1}{2}$oz
20g	$\frac{3}{4}$oz
30g	1oz
35g	1$\frac{1}{4}$oz
40g	1$\frac{1}{2}$oz
55g	2oz
60g	2$\frac{1}{4}$oz
65g	2$\frac{1}{2}$oz
75g	3oz
80g	3$\frac{1}{4}$oz
90g	3$\frac{1}{2}$oz
115g	4oz
125g	4$\frac{1}{2}$oz
150g	5oz
175g	6oz
180g	6$\frac{1}{4}$oz
200g	7oz
225g	8oz
250g	9oz
275g	10oz
300g	10$\frac{1}{2}$oz
325g	11$\frac{1}{2}$oz
350g	12oz
375g	13oz
400g	14oz
425g	15oz
450g	1 lb

Volume

30ml	1fl oz
50ml	2fl oz
75ml	2$\frac{1}{2}$fl oz
85ml	3fl oz
100ml	3$\frac{1}{2}$fl oz
125ml	4fl oz
150ml	5fl oz ($\frac{1}{4}$ pint)
175ml	6fl oz
200ml	7fl oz ($\frac{1}{3}$ pint)
225ml	8fl oz
240ml	8$\frac{1}{2}$fl oz
250ml	9fl oz
300ml	10fl oz ($\frac{1}{2}$ pint)
350ml	12fl oz
400ml	14fl oz
450ml	15fl oz ($\frac{3}{4}$ pint)
500ml	18fl oz
600ml	20fl oz (1 pint)

Measurements

5mm	$\frac{1}{4}$in
1cm	$\frac{1}{2}$in
2cm	$\frac{3}{4}$in
2.5cm	1in
3cm	1$\frac{1}{4}$in
4cm	1$\frac{1}{2}$in
5cm	2in
6.5cm	2$\frac{1}{2}$in
7cm	2$\frac{3}{4}$in
7.5cm	3in
9cm	3$\frac{1}{2}$in
10cm	4in
11cm	4$\frac{1}{2}$in
12.5cm	5in
15cm	6in
18cm	7in
20cm	8in
23cm	9in

Nutritional Tips

PROTEIN
We recommend eating 70–80g per day for women and 90–100g for men. Protein is needed for the healthy function of your biological systems, including producing hormones, repair and maintaining a healthy immune system. It also makes meals more filling. As well as using the treats in this book as ways to increase your protein intake, here are some other good sources of protein that you could add to your meal, or serve alongside the Bird Seed Crackers on page 86.

Cheese Top-Ups
1 tbsp grated cheese, around 10g
   (41 cals, 2.5g protein)
20g Parmesan, grated (82 cals, 7g protein)
30g Cheddar (124 cals, 7.5g protein)
50g feta (124 cals, 7.5g protein)
30g halloumi, sliced, lightly fried in 1 tsp olive
   oil for 4–5 minutes (130 cals, 6g protein)
50g soft cheese, such as Brie
   (171 cals, 10g protein)

Other Top-Ups
40g Greek yoghurt (53 cals, 2g protein)
2 tsp sesame seeds, around 10g
   (63 cals, 2g protein)
Handful of nuts, approx. 10g total weight,
   e.g. walnuts, pecans, hazelnuts
   (71 cals, 2g protein)
15g flaked almonds (95 cals, 4g protein)
1 medium boiled egg (78 cals, 7g protein)

HEALTHY COMPLEX CARBS
Ditch white flour and embrace complex carbs instead, which contain important nutrients and are an excellent source of fibre.

Healthy wholegrains
We've used spelt flour, buckwheat flour, oats and ground almonds instead of white flour in all our treats.

Clever Swap – If you purée fruit and pour it into an ice-cube tray, you can freeze it to make little morsels of sweetness. Use the cubes to add a hint of sweetness, if you need it, instead of reaching for sugar.

Index

ACKNOWLEDGEMENTS

Thanks to such a brilliant team for making this happen with good humour and time to spare!

Recipe writer: A huge thank you to Kathryn Bruton for your good humour, organisation, creative flair, wise inspiration and attention to detail – it's a privilege working with you.

Recipe tester: Caroline Barton, thank you for making testing fun, and for finessing recipes, while also providing excellent nutritional advice.

Nutritional analysis: Fiona Hunter, thanks for the extensive analyses that ensure the nutritional balance is as it should be.

Project editor: Jo Roberts-Miller, thank you for being so calm, super-efficient and incredibly effective, as well as having such great judgment.

Design, art direction and photography: Smith & Gilmour, we just love your clean, colourful and engaging images and design – spot on. Thank you too for delivering a fabulously stylish and appealing cover design as always.

Food styling: Phil Mundy, the wonderful bright, fun and enticing images are superb.

Production: Emily Noto, thank you for pulling things together!

Marketing and sales: A huge thanks to an excellent team, including Caroline Brown, Marianne Laidlaw, Matthew Grindon, Katherine Stroud, and especially Antonia Byrne for her patience and wise Instagram advice.

Publisher: Joanna Copestick, a pleasure to work with you and thank you for your encouragement, and for making it all come together.

Commissioning editor: Helena Sutcliffe, I can't thank you enough for your efficient, calm and positive approach. You make it all look deceptively easy, which I'm sure it isn't!

Fiona Hazard and Jacquie Brown: Thank you for your support. It's fantastic to have the brilliant Australian team with us too!

Anna Bond: my gratitude to you for all your support, wise words and for gently steering the tiller.

And most of all I send my love to my inspiration Michael and my family.

DR CLARE BAILEY, wife of Michael Mosley, has supported hundreds of patients during her medical career to lose weight, reduce their blood sugars and put their diabetes into remission. She is the author of *The 8-Week Blood Sugar Diet Recipe Book*, *The Clever Guts Diet Recipe Book*, *The Fast 800 Recipe Book*, *The Fast 800 Easy* and *The Fast 800 Keto Recipe Book*.

Instagram @drclarebailey

KATHRYN BRUTON is a recipe writer, developer and food stylist who contributes to the UK's bestselling cookbooks and leading food magazines. She is the author of her own bestselling series of low-calorie, high-nutrition cookbooks and now collaborates with leading authors to curate dynamic, must-cook recipes.

Instagram @kathryn_bruton